MOVE TO LIVE MORE

A Guide for Parents
and Caregivers to Help
Their Kids Move More
and Feel Better

Amy Bantham, DrPH

Move to Live More
A Guide for Parents and Caregivers to Help Their Kids Move More and Feel Better

Copyright © 2024 by Amy Bantham, DrPH

All rights reserved. No part of this book may be reproduced or transmitted in any form or by any means without written permission of the author.

ISBN 978-82-18-30877-4

Published by:
Move to Live More, LLC
Somerville, MA 02144

For Ben, Owen, Anna & Zoe

Contents

1. Introduction 1
2. Whole Child Health 7

Section I   Physical Health 13
3. Physical Health 15
4. Obesity 21
5. Physical Fitness 27
6. Physical Literacy 33

Section II   Mental Health 39
7. Mental Health 41
8. Play 47
9. Fun 53
10. Positivity 59

Section III   Academic Development 65
11. Academic Development 67
12. Leadership 75
13. Teamwork 81
14. Managing Risk 89

Section IV   The Role of Parents and Caregivers 95
15. The Role of Parents and Caregivers 97
16. Access 105
17. Family Support 111
18. Role Models 117
19. Balance 123
20. Conclusion 129

About the Author 133
Endnotes 135

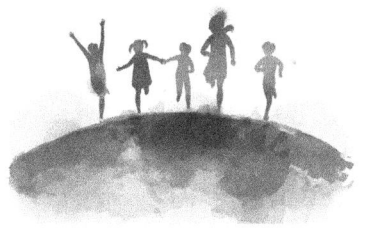

CHAPTER 1

Introduction

I'M AN UNLIKELY fitness professional. I wasn't an athlete or even a particularly active kid. Oftentimes, I was happiest when tucked away in a corner with a stack of books. I hated gym class. I still shudder when I remember my failed attempts to climb the rope, and that sinking feeling I'd get as captains picked teams—the loud, fast boys picked first; the quiet, bookish girls picked last. It was a popularity contest that I never won.

I had a brief stint running track and cross country in middle and high school. I enjoyed the camaraderie of being on a team and the feeling I experienced when I beat my previous best time in a race. But I was sidelined by injuries from pounding the pavement during practice. My running career was over before it ever really began.

Really, I didn't discover my love of movement until college. My roommates and I would head to a Friday afternoon group exercise class to close out a hard week of exams and papers. The class was led by an instructor who would captivate and motivate a gym full of college students for sixty minutes of heart-thumping aerobics. Hundreds of pairs of eyes were on her; hundreds of bodies mimicked her every movement. She was part performer, part coach, part cheerleader. She was able to whip the room into a frenzy of excitement, positive energy, and non-stop movement. I wanted to learn how to do that.

It took a while for me to step into the fitness professional role, and even longer to *own* it. At my first job after college, many of us would troop down to the company gym at lunchtime for an aerobics class. We worked long days, and it was a much-needed break. It was convenient, inexpensive, and fun.

One day, the instructor pulled me aside and said, "I think you should become an instructor. You would be great at it."

I was flattered. Though, I wondered what she had seen in me. Was it my form and technique? Was it the way I moved to the music? Was it my potential to lead a room full of fellow exercise enthusiasts? With my confidence growing and my interest piqued, I enrolled in an instructor training program. Every weekend for the next several months, I learned the theory of how to be a fitness professional. I studied textbooks—from anatomy to choreography, to programming. And then I put all that book knowledge into practice by running my classmates through mock classes—leading, cueing, and motivating. After sitting for and passing my certification exam, I became a fitness professional... on paper.

It was hard for me to move from being a fitness professional "in theory" to a *practicing* fitness professional. I still had doubts that the quiet, bookish girl picked last in gym class had what it would take to lead a room full of people in exercise. I'd just started graduate school and had little time. I was also a little bit embarrassed to admit to my fellow classmates that I was an aerobics instructor. At the time, the title still conjured up images of Jane Fonda, thongs, and leg warmers.

INTRODUCTION

After years of teaching group exercise, however, it has become one of the most important ways that I identify myself professionally. Today, I can proudly say that I am a Doctor of Public Health, a CEO, a physical activity researcher, and a fitness professional. My research and consulting work gets entire communities moving. It has a large-scale impact but can at times feel far removed from everyday people's lives. Leading exercise classes keeps me grounded in the field and allows me to see firsthand the impact that movement can have on helping people feel better and feel stronger.

One of the most important ways that I identify myself is as a mother of three children—a 13-year-old son and twin 11-year-old daughters. My children are a daily reminder of the impact that movement can have on people's mood, outlook, and ability to manage stress. When they are moving, their worries and fears slip away and they are at their most confident and joyful. I became involved with community physical activity advocacy because of them.

Children need at least sixty minutes of physical activity every day. They can get this activity at different touch points throughout the day—walking to school, recess, physical education (PE) class, after-school programs, weekend sports games, and family time are some examples that come to mind. I can help ensure that my kids are getting enough physical activity during the time that I spend with them or arrange for them, but I have little control over the eight hours they spend at school and in after-school programming each weekday.

For years they attended an elementary school without a gym or a cafeteria, so if they were truly going to be physically active, they needed to be outside. However, increasingly—and alarmingly—they told me stories of entire days spent indoors with juggling and hall bowling as their only physical activity. One year for his birthday, my son received an activity tracker as a gift. I remember how excited he was to wear it to school. I also remember how alarmed I was to see that after a week, he had averaged only about 4,000 steps per day (and that included the walk to and from school). Comparing this with the 12,000 to 16,000 steps per day that active boys between the ages of six to eleven are expected to get, I was very concerned.

I met with school personnel about the lack of physical activity, but nothing changed. Frustrated but undeterred, I started picking my kids up from their after-school program early one day a week, and that's how "Dr. B's Activity Hour" was born. On those days my kids and I would spend at least sixty minutes participating in active games and other activities together at a local park. But it was only one day a week. I wondered about the children whose parents and caregivers couldn't do this.

I joined our city's wellness committee, and we spent years advocating for, and ultimately gaining approval for a wellness policy that encouraged more physical activity—particularly outdoor physical activity—in our city's schools. But implementing the policy was challenging. We weren't able to have the impact that I had hoped in getting kids moving more during the school day. And then COVID-19 hit. In one fell sweep—and for an entire year—my kids and their classmates lost access to almost all their school-related physical activity opportunities.

The COVID-19 pandemic was a very dark time for families everywhere. Families struggled with job and income loss, disrupted schedules, remote and hybrid schooling, learning loss, lack of social connectedness, fears about illness, finding childcare, balancing home and work life, accessing support services that schools provided, and much more. For our family, movement has always been our one bright light. My kids are at their happiest when they are playing soccer, frisbee, or tag outside after dinner. They are magical on the soccer pitch—one of the few safe spaces from their worries and fears.

I have spent the past twenty-five years pursuing my life's purpose—helping people live healthier, happier, longer, more active

INTRODUCTION

lives. Along the way I have learned a few things about motivation and behavior change, and the connection between movement and physical, mental, social, and emotional health. I have learned from my own experience. I have also learned from thought leaders who are knocking down silos and stigmas to collaborate, communicate, and innovate their way to a solution for physical inactivity.

I have learned that movement is better than medicine. It improves kids' physical health, mental health, social emotional health, focus, and concentration. We are just beginning to understand the devastating toll of the pandemic on kids' health. We already know, though, that we are in desperate need of solutions. Movement is an important tool in our toolbox. This book is made up of lessons learned and is intended to serve as a guide for parents and caregivers to get their whole families moving to feel better and feel stronger. Move, to live more. Move, for a healthier life. Move, for a happier life.

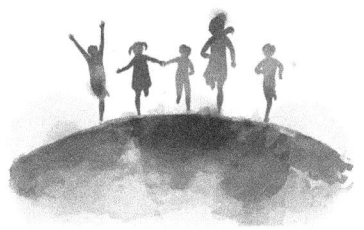

CHAPTER 2

Whole Child Health

THE "WHOLE CHILD" approach to children's health, education, and development is child-centered. This means that the number one priority focus is the child. The goal is for the child to feel healthy, safe, challenged, supported, and engaged.[1]

Children's health, education, and development are not influenced in just one setting, but rather in multiple settings. The Centers for Disease Control and Prevention (CDC) Whole School, Whole Community, Whole Child (WSCC) framework addresses child health in schools, in communities, and at home.[2]

In addition, children's health, education, and development is influenced by multiple factors, including teachers, public health professionals, and families. Their common cause is helping children achieve their best health and learning outcomes.

Health is defined as not just the absence of disease, but a state of complete physical, mental, and social well-being.[3] Whole Child health focuses on all aspects of a child's health, education, and development. It is multi-dimensional, and the three dimensions that we will refer to throughout this book—and which form the basis of the first three sections of the book—include: physical health; mental, social, and emotional health; and focus, concentration, and academic development.

Physical health is the condition of the body. Maintaining a healthy weight, eating a balanced diet, being physically active, and getting enough sleep all influence physical health. In turn, physical health and the condition of the body have a strong interrelationship with mental health and the condition of the mind.

Mental health is mental or psychological health and well-being that enables people to cope with life stresses.[4] Social and emotional health is the ability to understand and manage our emotions and to form social connections and relationships.[5] The Collaborative for Academic, Social, and Emotional Learning (CASEL) social and emotional learning framework revolves around five core social and emotional competencies, which include: self-awareness; self-management; responsible decision-making; relationship skills; and social awareness.[6]

Physical and mental health are deeply intertwined with focus, concentration, and academic development. Children who eat breakfast and generally have healthy dietary behaviors have better classroom outcomes, relating both to academic performance and discipline.[7] Children who are physically active have better grades, school attendance, cognitive performance, and classroom behavior.[8]

| Takeaways from Whole Child health

1. The "Whole Child" approach to children's health, education, and development is child-centered.

2. It is multi-dimensional, including physical health; mental, social, and emotional health; focus, concentration, and academic development.
3. Physical health, mental, social, and emotional health, and academic development are deeply intertwined.

How can parents and caregivers support Whole Child health?

As parents and caregivers, we want our children to reach their full potential. Fundamentally, we want our children to thrive—at home, at school, and throughout their lives. We see our role as giving them the foundation and building blocks they need to be well-rounded, healthy, and resilient children who become well-rounded, healthy, and resilient adults.

During the pandemic, the School Committee in my city held meetings where parents and caregivers could testify before Committee members. Our schools were remote for over a year and, often, the testimony at Committee meetings was from parents and caregivers advocating for a return to in-person schooling. I recall one parent who was concerned that her child not only was not thriving doing Zoom school, but was "withering."

That image really stuck with me. Just as plants need certain things to grow, our children need certain things to thrive. Without these things, our children can "wither."

Parents and caregivers can help our children thrive by taking a Whole Child approach to their health. We need to help our children meet their physical health needs by providing food and water. We can encourage them to sleep, move, and get outdoors.

We must also help our kids achieve their mental, social, and emotional health needs. It wasn't until the pandemic—when my children were homebound and computer-bound, alone and away from their friends—that I realized the extent to which they needed movement and social connectedness to thrive.

It was not just my children or specific to my city. This was an issue that was pervasive throughout the United States. A review of state school reopening plans in all fifty states and the District of Columbia compared the plans to the ten components of the WSCC model. The ten components are: PE and physical activity; nutrition environment and services; health education; social and emotional climate; physical environment; health services; counseling, psychological and social services; employee wellness; community involvement; and family engagement.

The review noted that twenty-three states established policy and practice requirements related to physical environment, such as cleaning, disinfecting, masking, and social distancing in their school reopening plans. In contrast, fewer than ten states included requirements related to non-physical health and wellness support for students, including social and emotional climate and counseling, and psychological and social services. In general, reviewers found that the plans had gaps in specific guidance for how schools should support the Whole Child during the pandemic, particularly their mental, social, and emotional health needs.[9]

How can parents and caregivers work with schools on Whole Child health?

Action for Healthy Kids is a national nonprofit organization with a mission to make schools healthy places where kids thrive. It began twenty years ago as an advocacy organization. Healthy eating and physical activity were the cornerstones of its work, as it sought to raise awareness of the childhood obesity epidemic.

The organization has expanded to include a national network of 50,000 schools. Its focus has also expanded to include mental, social, and emotional health programming, called "ConnectEd." It also continues to offer its core nutrition and physical activity and active play programming, called "NourishEd" and "EnergizEd," respectively.

The CEO of Action for Healthy Kids, Rob Bisceglie, sees the Whole Child approach as the basis for its entire model. According to Rob, "The only way I know to approach that issue is from a Whole Child perspective. I have spent 15 years studying and experiencing this, I see no other way. All the issues that kids face are intertwined. You can't separate them out and say, Oh, we're gonna deal with the nutrition or the physical activity, or make sure that they have a connection to a school nurse or make sure that they have mental health support. It is all those things, it's the only way to do it."[10]

Action for Healthy Kids recognizes that school and home are the two most important settings in a child's life. It factors in that children spend part of their day in school and part of their day and their entire summer out of school. Accordingly, it intentionally fosters development of strong family-school partnerships.

Its guidance for parents and caregivers to develop these strong family-school partnerships includes:

1. Visiting the school to learn about the school's culture and practices related to student health.
2. Asking questions of school leaders about how they would like families to support student health.
3. Gathering perspectives and ideas from other families to understand the school community's needs and concerns.
4. Using their voice as a parent or caregiver to share their needs and concerns.
5. Bringing a collaborative, solution-focused mindset to student health.[11]

Rob Bisceglie recommends that parents and caregivers be leaders and advocates themselves; and find these kinds of role models at their child's school. He believes that these leaders and advocates are in every school in the United States and are the key to change. "I have not seen a school that doesn't understand, intellectually, anyway, the importance of health and well-being for their kids... Our educators are absolutely, positively aware of this. The real problem is, it's an issue of priorities. It is stacked up against all these other issues that we have now lumped down to our schools. And so, I think it's really important that we identify those school leaders who are passionate about health and well-being and work with them to build school health teams."[12]

> **TIPS FOR PARENTS AND CAREGIVERS**
>
> 1. Take a Whole Child approach to your child's health, education, and development.
>
> 2. Prioritize physical health, mental, social, emotional health, and academic development; and recognize how interconnected these three dimensions are.
>
> 3. Recognize that children need to learn the building blocks of whole health, including nutrition and activity habits, that will help them thrive as children and adults.

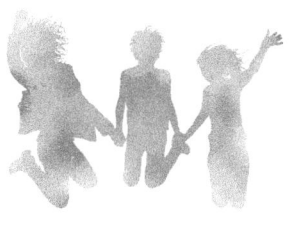

SECTION I

Physical Health

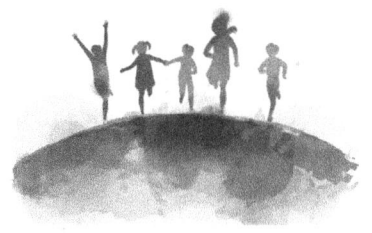

CHAPTER 3

Physical Health

PHYSICAL HEALTH IS one of the three dimensions of Whole Child health that this book covers, and the focus of the first section of the book. Physical activity contributes to physical health, but it is not the only contributor. Additionally, physical health is impacted by eating a balanced diet, getting enough sleep, and avoiding risky behaviors.[13]

This book does touch on these other influences on the condition of the body. However, its primary focus is the linkage between physical activity and physical health, physical activity and mental, social and emotional health, and physical activity and academic development.

Physical activity has numerous physical health benefits for children and adolescents.[14] It impacts the heart, lungs, bones, and muscles. It improves aerobic fitness, muscular fitness, and bone health. It also helps regulate body weight and reduce body fat. Body composition is the most used indicator to assess and evaluate physical health in children, and Body Mass Index (BMI) is the most common method to assess body composition.[15]

Levels of physical activity in childhood predict physical activity levels in adulthood.[16] In other words, children who are physically active tend to grow up to be adults who are physically active. On the flip side, children who are not physically active tend to grow up to be adults who are not physically active.

The levels of physical activity in children are concerning, and even more concerning in adolescents, as physical activity levels drop as children age. Whereas 42% of U.S. children between the ages of 6 and 11 meet physical activity guidelines, only 15.3% of 12 to 17-year-olds do.[17] Further, only 20% of adolescents meet physical activity guidelines globally.[18]

Physical activity levels are trending downward. In 2007, almost 30% of U.S. children between the ages of 6 and 17 met physical activity guidelines, and this decreased to 20% by 2019.[19] The COVID-19 pandemic exacerbated these downward trends. Globally, children's physical activity levels decreased by 17 minutes per day during the COVID-19 pandemic compared with pre-pandemic levels.[20] Similarly, U.S. children moved less and sat more during the pandemic.[21]

Physical fitness and physical activity are often confused or mistakenly used interchangeably. Physical fitness is the set of attributes or characteristics people have or achieve that relate to the ability to perform physical activity.[22] It includes a number of components, including cardiorespiratory fitness, muscular fitness (strength and endurance), motor fitness, metabolic fitness, and morphological fitness (body composition).[23]

Physical fitness levels are declining over time. Approximately 42% of 12-15-year-old children had adequate cardiorespiratory fitness in 2012. This earned us a C- in physical fitness according to the 2022 U.S. Report Card on Physical Activity for Children and

Youth (and highlighting the need for more recent national data than 2012).[24]

Obesity in children is defined as a BMI at or above the 95th percentile of the CDC BMI-for-age growth charts.[25] Approximately 1 in 5 U.S. children have obesity, which translates into 14.7 million children across the country.[26] During the first several months of the COVID-19 pandemic (March-November 2020), rates of BMI increase among children approximately doubled compared to the years prior to the pandemic (January 2018-February 2020).[27] Moreover, children who already had overweight or obesity prior to the pandemic experienced significantly higher rates of BMI increase during the pandemic than did those with healthy weight.[28]

Obesity in childhood predicts obesity in adulthood. In fact, children who have obesity are five times more likely to have obesity as adults.[29] Thus, early intervention is key. In early 2023, the American Academy of Pediatrics issued new clinical practice guidelines on the evaluation and treatment of obesity in children and adolescents. It prioritized early intervention and recommended against "watchful waiting" or delayed treatment.[30] The guidance included recommendations to refer children with obesity for intensive health behavior and lifestyle treatment. It also recommended medical and surgical interventions for children as young as 12, which generated a great deal of controversy.[31]

▌Takeaways from physical health

1. Physical activity has numerous physical health benefits for children and adolescents, impacting the heart, lungs, bones, and muscles.
2. Physical activity and obesity in childhood predicts physical activity and obesity in adulthood.

3. Physical activity levels are trending downward, and obesity levels are trending upward. Both trends were accelerated by the COVID-19 pandemic.

How can parents and caregivers help our kids experience the physical health benefits of movement?

Ken Rose is the Chief of CDC's Physical Activity and Health Branch in the Division of Nutrition, Physical Activity and Obesity. Ken and his team lead the Active People, Healthy Nation™ initiative, with a goal to help 27 million Americans become more physically active by the year 2027.[32] Active People, Healthy Nation seeks to move approximately 2 million young people toward meeting the minimum aerobic physical activity guideline.[33] According to Ken, "[the initiative] really is about creating a movement. We work with partners across sectors to make physical activity accessible to all communities. Everyone has a role to play to help physical activity become a way of life in the United States."[34]

The Physical Activity Guidelines for Americans were issued in 2008 and updated in 2018. They recommended children and adolescents ages 6 through 17 years do 60 minutes or more of moderate-to-vigorous physical activity daily, including aerobic, muscle-strengthening, and bone-strengthening activity.[35]

Move Your Way® is a campaign that promotes the recommendations of the Physical Activity Guidelines for Americans. The campaign recognizes the important role parents and caregivers play in helping our children experience all the health benefits of physical activity, and in meeting the recommended levels of physical activity. Specifically, there are fact sheets and posters, videos, interactive tools, stories, and sample social media messages written for parents and caregivers.[36]

How can parents and caregivers talk to our kids about physical activity and physical health?

Parents and caregivers can serve as facilitators to our kids getting enough physical activity. We can model physically active behavior. We can create a culture of physical activity in the home, by being physically active together with our children. We can sign our kids up for sports and active classes. We can share information about the health benefits of being physically active. We can provide words of encouragement and support.

Language matters. Parents and caregivers can talk about physical activity in terms of overall health, not weight loss. If their child brings up the issue of weight, parents and caregivers can use strategies recommended by the STOP Obesity Alliance and the Alliance for a Healthier Generation, as outlined in their conversation guide for talking to children.[37] Parents and caregivers are encouraged to: 1) thank their child for sharing their feelings; 2) ask open-ended questions so their child can express their feelings; 3) identify that weight is a matter of health, not looks; 4) acknowledge the challenges to being healthy, but also the benefits of better health; and 5) offer to work together to be healthier together.

Parents and caregivers can also talk about physical activity in terms of fun. Move Your Way encourages parents and caregivers to focus on fun, with a reminder to "make fun the name of the game." As Ken Rose also puts it, "it is important for people to see that physical activity can be fun. It can be as simple as going for a walk with friends or dancing to your favorite song. Physical activity plays an important part in improving our recreational quality of life."[38]

TIPS FOR PARENTS AND CAREGIVERS

1. Encourage your children to get 60 minutes of physical activity per day, including aerobic, muscle-strengthening, and bone-strengthening activity.

2. Talk about physical activity in terms of overall health, not weight loss.

3. Talk about physical activity in terms of fun, togetherness, and quality of life.

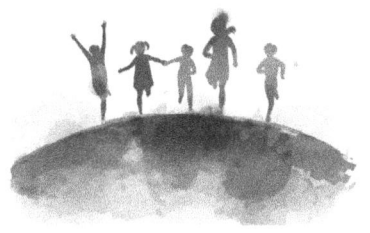

CHAPTER 4

Obesity

Innovative Initiatives Helping Children with Obesity - Quality, Daily PE

DR. DANIEL FULHAM O'Neill is an orthopedic surgeon, sports medicine doctor, and sport psychologist with a mission to revolutionize and rebrand PE. He authored a book called, *Survival of the Fit: How Physical Education Ensures Academic Achievement and a Healthy Life*, which envisions a world where every child has access to quality PE in school every day.

He was spurred into action by the number of children in his personal life—as well as his professional life through his practice—who were struggling with obesity and fitness. He has seen a huge shift over time in children's level and type of activity. He used to see children who were burned out from doing too many activities and sports. Now he sees children who are burned out from too much sedentary social media time.

This shift is heading us in the wrong direction. "It's this aircraft carrier that just can't seem to get turned around. And again, this is not some secret thing. Everybody… knows that we have a problem in this country with obesity, with fitness."[39]

Dr. O'Neill feels a great sense of urgency to address the problem of childhood obesity and lack of physical fitness. He notes the impact on children's lifespan and quality of life. In fact, he cites evidence that this generation of children will be the first generation in history who have a shorter lifespan than their parents.

The COVID-19 pandemic revealed the high stakes of having such an unhealthy youth population. "The only young people who died from this virus were unhealthy kids, or kids with obesity."[40]

Dr. O'Neill defines physical identity as the innate human drive to move, play and explore. He sees this instinctive drive being eroded by constant screen time-based sedentary behavior. He calls out age seven in particular as the tipping point when physical identity lapses and becomes more difficult to reclaim. And he sees quality, daily PE beginning at an early age and continuing throughout school years as a way to counteract this erosion. He believes that it needs to start in kindergarten, it needs to be every day, and it needs to be quality instruction where kids are moving every minute of the PE class. The end result is that "[children] have their physical identity, [and] they know for at least 180 days a year they are going to be expected to get their heart rates up."[41]

He recognizes that everyone needs to be a part of the PE revolution and that advocacy needs to come from as many different stakeholders as possible. Because they are up against a powerful foe. He points a finger at the technology companies headquartered in Silicon Valley in California as culpable in developing technology that addicts children to screens. "But what we're trying to do as parents is fight Silicon Valley to not addict our children to screen time. And that is a fight we are losing."[42] He calls on parents and caregivers to fight back against processed foods and screens, and the entities that make them such a large part of our children's lives.

Takeaways from Quality, Daily PE as an Innovative Initiative Helping Children with Obesity

1. Children spend too much time in sedentary activity and not enough time in quality, daily PE.
2. Lack of quality, daily PE is having significant implications for children's obesity and physical fitness levels.
3. Quality, daily PE is a way for parents and caregivers to guard against too much sedentary screen time.

What can parents and caregivers do about obesity?

Parents and caregivers may become concerned about obesity if there is a visible increase in their child's size. There may be a noticeable change in eating patterns and activity levels. Healthcare providers may flag a change in their growth charts at their annual physicals.

My friends with children who have obesity share their struggles. They often feel very protective of their children and are concerned that their children will be made fun of by their peers. They worry about the long-term consequences for their children's health. They wrestle with making too much of an issue of it, worried that it could drive their children away from activity instead of toward it.

They often feel enormous pressure to solve the problem themselves. Yet, children spend eight or more hours a day in school. We as parents and caregivers can only control the amount of activity that our children do during out-of-school hours and even then, we don't have full control.

In fact, parents and caregivers often have the most success when we give our children control over their activity choices. We can offer a variety of options, and then explore with our children the type of activity that appeals to them the most. For example, if our children mention liking frisbee, we can make a standing date with them to toss a frisbee outside. If that goes well, we can enroll them in ultimate frisbee programs.

Parents and caregivers can talk about the activity as something to do for fun, not something to do for weight loss. Our children are more likely to have fun doing an activity if their friends do it as well. It can also be a whole family activity.

Another thing parents and caregivers can do is focus our time and attention on getting our children more activity before and after school and during weekends and evenings. For in-school activity, over which we have minimal control, we can join forces with other parents and caregivers to advocate for more PE, recess, and active classrooms.

What can parents and caregivers do about technology and sedentary time?

The issue of technology and sedentary time is a really challenging one for parents and caregivers. During the COVID-19 pandemic, children who were doing online school were sitting in front of screens all day. Even children who had minimal or no screen time before the pandemic had at least six to eight hours of screen time a day with online school. My daughter really suffered from the constant exposure to the blue light given off by the computer screen. She had crippling headaches that were moderately improved with special glasses, but only disappeared once she returned to in person school.

Moreover, parents and caregivers who were desperate for "safe" ways for our children to gather with their peers would allow them to play online games. I weighed the hours of additional screen time against the need for social connection, and the need for social connection won out. My children started playing online games with their school friends during the pandemic, and I was happy they had that outlet. They balanced it with outdoor time with friends each day after online school ended.

Parents and caregivers juggling working from home and overseeing online school often resorted to additional screen time for our children in the evenings. It was often the only way to catch up on missed work. My husband and I found it very difficult to work an eight-hour day while also making sure our three children logged into and out of online school at the appropriate times, not to mention helping them with schoolwork and homework. We would usually end up on our own computers after dinner, and we relaxed the rules about our children's screen time at night as well.

Parents and caregivers can help our children get out from behind their screens. We can set limits on our own use of screens, and apply them to our children's devices as well. For example, no devices at the family dinner table, or no devices after 8:00 pm. Family walks became very popular in our family during the pandemic. It was a way to unplug and have some type of connection to the outside world. Families can make sure we do one active thing together as a family, every day.

TIPS FOR PARENTS AND CAREGIVERS

1. Explore activity options with your children and help them choose one they are excited about.

2. Once your children find an activity they like and want to do, help them arrange to do it regularly with family or friends.

3. Focus on fun not weight loss.

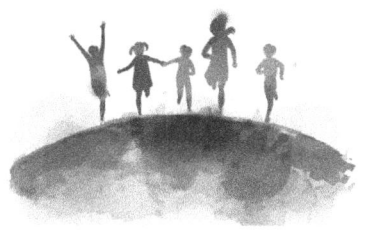

CHAPTER 5

Physical Fitness

Innovative Initiatives Helping Children with Physical Fitness - The Daily Mile

ELAINE WYLLIE WAS the principal at an elementary school in Scotland. She became very concerned about the physical fitness of her students when she noticed they were struggling to run the perimeter of the schoolyard. To address this, she put the students in charge of developing a program that would get them outside and moving daily. Created by children for children, The Daily Mile is exactly as it sounds—one mile, or approximately 15 minutes, per day when children run, jog, walk, or roll (for wheelchair users) around their school grounds, with their classroom teachers, as a class.

Elaine credits the universal appeal of The Daily Mile to the fact that it was invented by children, for children. She also believes that the reason that it "has been replicated across school cultures across climates across the world… is because The Daily Mile meets the needs of childhood—fun, fresh air, friends, freedom—and these needs are the same wherever you go."[43]

Studies demonstrate that children who participate in The Daily Mile improve their physical fitness. Specifically, the percentage of children classified as fit—as assessed by the 20-meter shuttle run test—increased by nine percentage points, or 51% to 60% from baseline to follow-up.[44] The original cohort of students responsible for creating The Daily Mile improved their physical fitness by measurable amounts, for example going on to win their national cross-country championships.

There is insufficient time spent on PE and sport during the school week to make most children fit, according to Elaine. In contrast, The Daily Mile uses time in the school week to make fitness accessible to all children, even those who are "a bit unathletic or a bit unfit."[45] As more and more children discover their "inner fit child,"[46] their worlds open up and they begin to enjoy PE and sport.

Studies have also demonstrated that The Daily Mile has a positive impact on children's mental fitness and well-being. In fact, children who participate in The Daily Mile improve their cognitive performance and well-being by seven percent, as measured by verbal memory, alertness, and mood.[47] Teachers who lead their classes in doing The Daily Mile report that students return to the classroom refreshed and ready to learn after having a chance to "reset" outdoors. (As an added bonus, teachers return to the classroom refreshed and ready to teach.)

Over ten years after The Daily Mile was developed by the Scottish elementary school, it has reached over 4 million children in more than 14,000 schools in 90 countries. But the problem of poor physical fitness is urgent and the reach needs to be even larger. According to Elaine, "[I]t's happening on our watch. And these children, the majority of children in the Western world, are overweight and unfit and that... is unacceptable. So, if not us, then who? If not now, then when?"[48]

Takeaways from The Daily Mile Helping Children with Physical Fitness

1. Children like to be asked for their ideas on how they can be active daily.
2. Children like to be active as a group with their peers and teachers.
3. Children (and grown-ups) benefit from having a chance to "reset" by being active outdoors.

What can parents and caregivers do about physical fitness?

It may be difficult for parents and caregivers to assess our children's physical fitness. The gold standard is a test that measures how well a child's heart and lungs send oxygen to the muscles during exercise. However, it is unlikely that parents and caregivers will take our children to have such a test administered in a lab or at a hospital, with all the necessary equipment. Instead, it is more likely that physical fitness might be assessed in a school setting using something like the shuttle run test, which requires minimal equipment.

What may be more visible to parents and caregivers is if our children are out-of-breath after walking up the stairs. We may also notice if they are having trouble keeping up with their siblings or peers when they are playing tag or hurrying to catch the bus.

Instilling healthy habits, including daily physical activity, starts in childhood. If we want our children to become fit, healthy adults, we need to help them become fit, healthy children who are active daily. Increasing physical activity generally improves physical fitness, and improved physical fitness generally improves health.

Parents and caregivers can help improve our children's physical fitness by ensuring that they have access to a wide range of activities.

Children can strengthen their hearts and lungs by walking, running, biking, swimming, and dancing, to name a few activities. Children can strengthen their muscles by climbing trees, using playground equipment, or climbing ropes. Children can strengthen their bones by skipping, playing hopscotch, or jumping rope.

Children—especially younger children—are not likely to be motivated by physical fitness as a goal. My 13-year-old son is reaching the age where physical fitness is part of his organized sports training. He finds increased speed and strength to be a tremendous motivator. However, I can't imagine my 11-year-old twin daughters rushing to do burpees and sit ups with "physical fitness" as the promised end result. Types of activities and motivators must be age appropriate.

Even for older children, we don't need to stand over them with a whistle to help them aspire to the goal of being physically fit. Rather, we can help them be active daily in order to feel better and stronger, with physical fitness as one of the many benefits of this active lifestyle.

How can parents and caregivers put children in charge of their own physical fitness?

Children are incredibly creative when coming up with activities that get them moving (and strengthen their hearts and lungs, muscles, and bones at the same time). Just as the children who created The Daily Mile were put in charge of developing a program that would get them outside and moving daily, parents and caregivers can put our children in charge of making up their own activities.

When I recognized that my children weren't getting enough physical activity in school, I picked them up once a week to take them to a nearby park for "Dr. B's Activity Hour." During the COVID-19 pandemic, I realized that many parents and caregivers might be struggling with getting kids outside and active, safely. So, I put "Dr. B's Activity Hour" down on paper and shared it with others, with the hope that many families might benefit from some socially distanced movement ideas.

The greatest sources of ideas for "Dr. B's Activity Hour" were my children. Every week, I would come armed with a few ideas and a few pieces of equipment. We would then take turns making up activities. Each child would be in charge of one activity, deciding every aspect of it: how many players, which moves, which equipment, what was and was not allowed, how it began, and how it ended. If they like competitive games, they would create competitive games. If they like cooperative games, they would create cooperative games.

I found that they were able to put together a variety of heart-, lung-, muscle-, and bone- strengthening activities that increased physical fitness. Yet, not once did we categorize the activities as heart-, lung-, muscle- or bone-strengthening. Not once did we discuss "physical fitness" as a goal. Not once did we say that these activities were training for organized sports, or anything besides an opportunity to move and to have fun.

Children like to jump, run, skip, and hop. They will have a lot of fun doing these things when they are with their peers (or even their siblings and parents and caregivers). They will take pride and feel empowered when given the great responsibility of creating activities for an entire group.

TIPS FOR PARENTS AND CAREGIVERS

1. Talk with your children about physical fitness as one of many benefits of being active daily.

2. Make it clear that physical fitness is important for all children—not just children who do organized sports. Physical fitness comes with being active daily.

3. Focus on fun not physical fitness.

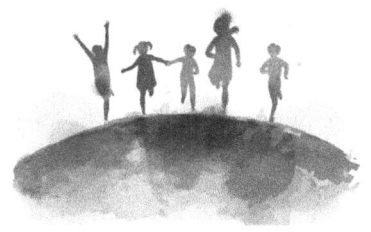

CHAPTER 6

Physical Literacy

Innovative Initiatives Helping Children with Physical Literacy—Making Health a Core Subject

CHUCK RUNYON IS the CEO and Co-Founder at Self-Esteem Brands, the parent company of Anytime Fitness, a fitness franchise with more than 4,700 gyms worldwide. Anytime Fitness works to "Make Healthy Happen" for all of its three million members through nutrition, physical activity, and mental health support, as well as affordable and accessible coaching.

Physical literacy is "the ability, confidence, and desire to be physically active for life."[49] Chuck sees a real lack of physical literacy in the adult population. The average adult does not know enough about how their body works, particularly when talking about implications for their health. For example, they tend to underestimate their caloric intake and overestimate their caloric expenditure.

He traces this lack of body intelligence and physical literacy to the educational system and declines in PE, sports, and extracurricular activities over the past 30 years. In the current educational system, math, reading, and science are valued but children are not learning how their bodies work. According to Chuck, "Just like we wouldn't tolerate poor grades in math, science or reading, we cannot tolerate poor grades in physical literacy."[50]

He believes that beginning in kindergarten and throughout college, health, physical activity, and nutrition should be taught—not as an elective, but as a core part of the curriculum. He finds this particularly important given the clear link between physical activity, mental acuity, and academic achievement. According to Chuck, "I think we have to reframe how we're teaching health and make sure that we show students how nutrition, fitness, activity, and recovery is a link towards mental acuity."[51]

When students graduate from school, they need to be equipped to succeed even while living in unhealthy environments. Chuck believes that understanding how their bodies work will help graduates be successful despite the lure of sedentary activities and high calorie, cheap meals. He invites each and every graduate to become the "CEO of their own health."[52]

Chuck is optimistic that the use of wearable technology will help make body intelligence and physical literacy more accessible to more people. The data collected from wearable technology can help people know more about how their bodies work. This knowledge, combined with support from fitness professionals, can help them set and achieve their health and fitness goals.

Takeaways from Making Health a Core Subject Helping Children with Physical Literacy

1. Health education needs to be prioritized as a core subject.
2. Physical literacy can be taught, and children who learn physical literacy will be better equipped to succeed in unhealthy environments.

3. Wearable technology can help make physical literacy more accessible to more people.

What can parents and caregivers do to promote physical literacy?

Parents and caregivers have a central role to play in developing physical literacy in our children. If we break the definition of physical literacy down into its three components—ability, confidence, and desire—parents and caregivers can impact each one.

Ability is competence in basic movement and sports skills. Just as parents and caregivers can help our children learn to read by teaching them letters and phonics—fundamental building blocks for reading—parents and caregivers can teach our children basic movement and sports skills in age- and developmentally-appropriate ways. For example, we can teach them how to catch balls of many different sizes and weights, and how to catch a softball hit by a bat. In addition, parents and caregivers can provide children access to the equipment they need to practice these skills. Finally, parents and caregivers can give them opportunities to learn these skills in a variety of different environments.

Confidence is belief in the ability to do the given physical activities. Parents and caregivers can boost our children's confidence by helping them practice basic movement and sports skills. With practice comes progress and with progress, confidence. Parents and caregivers can also boost our children's confidence by cheering them on and making them feel good about their mastery of the skills. Positive affirmations go a long way toward building confidence. Parents and caregivers can also ensure our children practice these skills with others who build them up rather than tearing them down. When my daughter was in the fourth grade, she played soccer on a team with fifth and sixth graders who were stronger, bigger, and faster, and who had been playing together longer. The entire experience could have eroded her confidence, but instead it boosted it. Why? Because her teammates always took the time to tell my daughter what she was doing right, and to comment on a nice pass or a well-timed block.

Desire is motivation to be physically active. Forcing children to practice basic movement and sports skills is a surefire way to demotivate them. It is similar to forcing them to do their homework or set the table. Instead, parents and caregivers can make skill development fun for our children by playing games—family games, games with friends, and unstructured active play. Children who are having fun and spending time with family and friends will be enthusiastic about doing it, and the skill development and mastery will happen as a byproduct, rather than being the main objective.

Parents and caregivers should not be expected to develop physical literacy in our children all by themselves. Development of physical literacy—through practice and mastery of basic movement and sports skills—is intended to be a primary outcome of physical and health education in schools. If parents and caregivers are not seeing that our children are receiving high quality, frequent, and effective physical and health education, they can join together with other parents and caregivers to advocate for it. When I saw that my kids weren't getting enough activity during the school day, I joined our District Wellness Committee as a parent volunteer. Rather than being the lone voice advocating for change at my school, I was one of many voices with the same goal of getting all the kids in our school district healthier and more active.

How can parents and caregivers use technology to develop physical literacy?

Wearable technology was the number one fitness trend in 2022, according to the American College of Sports Medicine Worldwide

Survey of Fitness Trends.[53] In the survey, wearables were defined as fitness trackers, smart watches, heart rate monitors, and GPS tracking devices. Their functionality includes counting steps and tracking heart rate, calories, sitting and sleep time, blood pressure, and respiratory rate.

As with adults, the best type of wearables for kids are ones that they know how to use and will wear consistently. I once sat on a panel focused on wearable technology with a number of experts in the field. We were asked about our own wearable preferences. One panelist held up an incredibly complicated smart watch that looked like it belonged in a laboratory. Another panelist showed arms with about ten activity trackers up to each elbow. I felt low tech in comparison with just one simple Fitbit on my wrist. But I stand by my choice because Fitbit works for me. It is simple and easy for me to use. My mother also had one for years, and with them we can be activity buddies.

I am not advocating that every parent run out and buy a complicated and expensive fitness tracker for their child. Cost is a barrier that makes wearables inaccessible to many families. In addition, children tend to lose them. My son dropped his Fitbit into the lining of one of the seats of our car and we have not been able to extricate it. Children also lose interest. One of my daughters has a Fitbit, but her interest in it goes in waves ranging from very interested and on her wrist every day to not at all interested and uncharged on her dresser.

That said, there is a role for wearables in the development of physical literacy. They can positively impact all three components of physical literacy—ability, confidence, and desire. They can help children track how much and what they are doing and how they are progressing, and they can do it in a way that is fun and motivating.

TIPS FOR PARENTS AND CAREGIVERS

1. Focus on the fun, not the skills development.
2. Boost your children's confidence through practice and positive reinforcement.
3. Consider wearables as one tool to support ability, confidence, and the desire to be physically active.

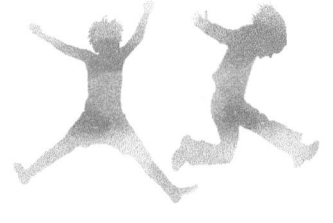

SECTION II

Mental Health

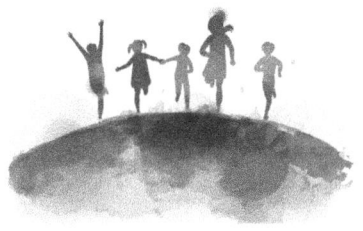

CHAPTER 7

Mental Health

MENTAL HEALTH IS the second of the three dimensions of Whole Child health that this book covers. This section is devoted to mental health and the intersection between physical activity and mental health.

Mental health refers to our emotional, psychological, and social well-being.[54] It is so integral to health that there is no health without mental health.[55] For years, we talked about mental health and physical health as if they were separate things. But increasingly, the focus has shifted to the interconnectedness of the mind and the body. There is a growing recognition that a healthy body and a healthy mind are both necessary for a healthy person.

Kids' emotions and behaviors are influenced by mental health. It influences how they feel about themselves, and how they feel about others. It impacts how they cope with stress and adversity and regulate their own emotions. Mental health also impacts how children act toward themselves, and how they interact with others.

It's no secret that we are facing a youth mental health crisis. Not a day goes by when we don't see a headline telling us what we see in front of our eyes every single day.

"The Kids Are Not Alright!" proclaim these headlines.

"We know!" we as parents and caregivers respond. We see that our kids are sad, stressed, and worried. Their worries are big and ever present and seem even bigger than when we were kids.

What or who is to blame for the youth mental health crisis? Fingers are often pointed at the COVID-19 pandemic, as kids experienced collective trauma. They are months, even years, behind in their social and emotional development. Teachers who work with kids every day tell me their students were worried throughout the pandemic that they were going to get sick and die. They were also worried they were going to get their grandparents, parents, and siblings sick, and their loved ones were going to die. Those are big worries for little kids to have.

The COVID-19 pandemic did exacerbate the youth mental health crisis. A review of 29 studies including almost 81,000 children estimated that the global prevalence of depression and anxiety symptoms doubled during the pandemic.[56] In May 2020, 29% of parents with children and adolescents aged 5-18 said their children were "already experiencing harm" to their mental health because of social distancing and closures.[57]

In October 2020, one-third (31%) of U.S. parents with children aged 2-18 reported their child's emotional health was worse than before the COVID-19 pandemic.[58] Nearly two-thirds reported that their child had recently experienced a mental or emotional challenge—most commonly social isolation (23%), anxiety (22%), and trouble concentrating (20%).[59] Half of the teenagers surveyed in the study reported they had experienced mental or emotional health challenges in the past month—most commonly anxiety (28%), trouble concentrating (21%), and social isolation/loneliness (20%).[60]

In October 2021, the American Academy of Pediatrics, the American Academy of Child and Adolescent Psychiatry, and the Children's Hospital Association jointly declared a national state of emergency in child and adolescent mental health.[61] In December 2021, the U.S. Surgeon General issued a public advisory calling Americans' attention to the urgent issue of youth mental health. It cited a 51% increase in emergency room visits for suicide attempts for adolescent girls and a 4% increase for adolescent boys in early 2021 compared to 2019.[62]

The youth mental health crisis predated the COVID-19 pandemic, however. Between 2016 and 2019, 9.8% of children aged 3-17 years had been diagnosed with Attention Deficit Hyperactivity Disorder (ADHD), 9.4% with anxiety, 8.9% with behavior problems, and 4.4% with depression.[63] Between 2018 and 2019, 15.1% of adolescents aged 12-17 years had a major depressive episode, 36.7% had persistent feelings of sadness or hopelessness, and 18.8% seriously considered attempting suicide.[64]

What happened prior to the COVID-19 pandemic that impacted youth mental health? There is a lot of attention focused on 2012, when the number of Americans owning smartphones became the majority. Rates of happiness among U.S. teenagers, which increased between 1991 and 2011, declined in 2012 and after as rates of depression, suicidal ideation, and self-harm increased.[65] Smartphone and social media use displaced time spent on other activities. According to an annual nationally representative study, U.S teenagers who spend more time on electronic devices are less happy, while those who spend more time on most other activities, especially sleep and physical activity, are happier.[66]

What can we do about the youth mental health crisis? Currently, only about half of the children and adolescents with mental health disorders get treatment.[67] There are concerted efforts underway to address the shortage of mental health professionals who work with children and adolescents, but in addition to treatment, prevention is key. Sleep and physical activity, as well as nutrition, are important tools for us to have in our toolbox as we think about how we can help our kids.

Takeaways from mental health

1. Mental health includes emotional, psychological, and social well-being.
2. Mental health is so integral to health that there is no health without mental health.
3. The COVID-19 pandemic exacerbated a youth mental health crisis already underway, coinciding with smartphone and social media use.

How can physical activity help our kids' mental health?

There is a clear linkage between physical activity and mental health in kids. Kids who are physically active are less likely to have anxiety and depression. In fact, a study of 35,000 U.S. children and adolescents aged 6-17 years found that those who reported meeting the physical activity guidelines of 60 minutes or more per day were half as likely to have anxiety and depression as peers who did no physical activity. Moreover, some physical activity was better than none, as children who were physically active only one to three days a week still had lower rates of anxiety and depression.[68]

Physical activity in kids is linked to mental health into late adolescence and early adulthood as well. Depression scores at age 18 are lower for every additional 60 minutes per day of physical activity at ages 12, 14 and 16. Conversely, they are higher for every additional hour of sedentary behavior. Worryingly, by age 16, adolescents reported spending an average of 9 hours per day in sedentary behavior.[69]

It is important for us to get our kids moving for mental as well as physical health benefits. It is also important for us to get our kids to stop spending so much time sitting down. Sedentary behavior usually involves smartphone and social media use, which makes kids less happy. Moreover, it displaces activities that make kids feel happier, like sleep and physical activity. It can be really challenging to get our kids to unplug and move, but doing so could have a huge impact on their happiness.

How can parents and caregivers talk to our kids about physical activity and mental health?

We as parents and caregivers are worried about our children's mental health. In fact, parents placed mental health as our number one concern. Four out of ten U.S. parents with school-aged children say they are extremely or very worried that their children might struggle with anxiety or depression at some point.[70]

Because it is top of mind for us, we need to make it top of mind for our kids. Dr. Brendon Stubbs is one of the authors on the above referenced Kandola et al. study linking physical activity in kids with mental health as they grow up. According to Dr. Stubbs, "we all have mental health, and there [are] times where our mental health is out of sync, and many of us will have mental health symptoms or conditions at one point in our lives. And we all almost certainly know somebody right now who is struggling with a mental health diagnosis. So, it's only right that we're openly talking about mental health, and how we can help people."[71]

How do we bring up the topic of mental health with our children? We can check in with our kids regularly about how they are feeling. Encouraging them to come to us when they are angry, worried, or sad, as well as when they are happy. We can normalize mental health and talk about mental health the same way we might talk about physical health. We can also talk about positive mental health. Positive mental health indicators include affection, persistence, resilience, positivity, self-control, and curiosity.[72] We can try to model and reinforce these positive mental health indicators. And we can explain to our children that mental health exists on a continuum. Sometimes we have good mental health and sometimes we don't have quite as good mental health, just like sometimes we have good physical health and sometimes we don't have quite as good physical health.

In addition, we can emphasize that physical activity can be a coping strategy for stress. I am amazed by the night and day difference in my children before and after being physically active. For example, my son, stressed about an upcoming test during an entire car ride to soccer practice, he returned to the car after practice with a completely different demeanor—more focused, more positive, more relaxed. It is important for us to notice this, and to point this out to our children so that they can make the connection themselves.

TIPS FOR PARENTS AND CAREGIVERS

1. Make the connection for your kids between physical activity and positive feelings.

2. Get your kids to unplug from devices that keep them sitting for hours each day. Children and adolescents who spend more time on electronic devices are less happy, and those who spend more time on other activities, like sleep and physical activity, feel happier.

3. Talk about mental health as a continuum, and how there are good mental health days as well as not as good mental health days.

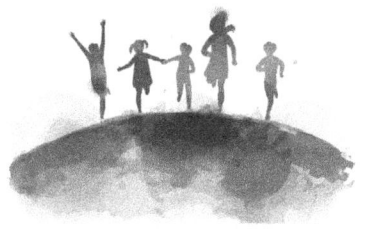

CHAPTER 8

Play

Innovative Initiatives Helping Children Move More - Reframing Exercise as Play

JANET OMSTEAD IS a health and behavior change coach, a self-described "play expert," and the Founder of the Play for Life system. Janet takes a playful approach to movement and sees play as "the freedom to move your body in any way that brings you joy, makes you sweat a little, and smile a lot."[73]

Janet completely reframes exercise as play. She finds that play feels like much less of a barrier for people struggling to find the time or motivation to go to the gym or do a hard workout. According to Janet, "play is a relatively low bar you can build on, and starting small and building up is what makes things sustainable. And it makes it less scary. Play just feels achievable."[74]

Children are the inspiration for much of Janet's philosophy toward movement and play. She admires their natural freedom of movement as she walks by playgrounds watching kids play tag, hang upside down from monkey bars, and make up creative games together. She notes that step counts and heart rate zones are probably the farthest things from their minds as they play and have fun.

Janet taps into her own inner child and coaches her clients to do the same. "[The] whole idea of playing and moving shouldn't have to stop just because we grow up… I think it's time we rediscover our inner kid and give ourselves permission to have fun."[75] Play and fun are key ingredients, which start a positive spiral of wanting to move more, eat better, and sleep better.

Playgrounds figure prominently in Janet's philosophy toward movement and play. In fact, the world is Janet's playground. She walks out the front door and her creative juices kick into gear about how she can move, and play, and find what brings her joy. She coaches her clients to view the world through a play lens as well—to eat well, manage stress in a way that makes sense to them, and to find activities that bring them joy.

Janet does not take a particularly prescriptive approach with her clients. Rather, she sees her role as providing support so that her clients can figure out what is going to work for them, in order to move the needle towards their own better health. Not magic potions or quick fixes, but small, consistent changes over time with play at the heart of it all.

Takeaways from Play Helping Children Move More

1. Children have a natural freedom of movement that allows them to play and have fun.
2. As they grow up, people lose their playful approach to movement.
3. Adults who give themselves permission to find our own inner child will be more successful in achieving their health goals.

How can parents and caregivers encourage a playful approach to movement?

Children have an innate instinct to play. Parents and caregivers can foster that innate instinct in our children at every stage of development. When my kids were very young, play was one of our top priorities in terms of how they spent their time. My children attended a preschool with a curriculum that supported an exploration of the world through play. It was the lens through which they (and we) saw everything.

Outdoor movement and exploration were emphasized at their preschool, with twice-a-day active outdoor time, rain or shine. After preschool ended each afternoon, my kids were at their happiest when we were outside playing. With three children born within three years, I wanted to be wherever they were happiest. Life was just too challenging otherwise. As my children started crawling, then walking, then running and jumping and climbing, playing actively at playgrounds was how we spent the majority of our time.

However, play became less and less of a priority as my children grew older. School became less about play and more about academic subjects. Sports became less about active play and more about training and competition. Play started to feel almost frivolous, at odds with serious academics or serious sports.

We had to intentionally re-introduce active play into our kids' lives. How did we do this? We took family walks after dinner. We would walk to a nearby apartment complex that was interesting because it had a koi pond in front of it. We would let the kids lead the way in exploring the complex and playing games on our way to and from it. In addition, we took family outings to a nearby park to kick a ball around. We also had family Olympics nights. After dinner we would head outside and plan the line-up of events, using whatever equipment we had available and choosing whatever activity the kids were in the mood for that evening. Badminton, soccer, and softball were favorites.

The COVID-19 pandemic was a mixed bag in its impact on our kids' active play. On one hand, the pandemic literally took the playground away. Nearby playgrounds, parks, and fields sat unused, wrapped in yellow police tape. We live in a very urban area and don't have a yard, so we rely heavily on public green spaces. One day, my family headed to a nearby park to play tag and soccer. We were sent home by an officer in a police car moving through the park with a bullhorn, telling all of us to leave immediately because the park was closed during the pandemic.

On the other hand, my daughters formed an outdoor "recess pod" with two other friends. Once parks reopened, they met in a local park every day for almost a year. They often drafted the supervising grown-ups into games of hide-and-seek or tag. They also developed their own incredibly creative games, which took advantage of the rock formations and walls in the park. They grew resilient by meeting up for "recess pod" every single day, even when it was raining or snowing.

Parents and caregivers can encourage our children to have a playful approach to movement by not standing in the way of their innate instinct to play, especially when they are young. When children are older and move away from play because of time constraints and different priorities, parents and caregivers can encourage them to meet up with friends for active play. We can also make it a core part of the time the family spends together.

How can parents and caregivers find our own inner child?

A key piece of encouraging a playful approach to movement in our kids is finding our own inner child. Often when I am spending time with my daughters, one of them will say, "Let's play tag, catch me." My immediate instinct is to say no. I am generally too tired, or too focused on work, or too conscious of the people around us who might not want to see a middle-aged woman chasing after her 11-year-old at high speed (or at least high speed for a middle-aged woman).

However, in order to find my own inner child, I need to remember the feelings of freedom that came with being uninhibited with movement when I was a child. I need to remember that I have the privilege of being able to move anywhere at any time, and not just inside the four walls of the health club where I teach group exercise every Wednesday morning. I need to put down my phone and look up from my computer, and engage with my children at the playground.

Parents and caregivers can model active play for our kids by playing actively ourselves. We can do it on our own or when we are with our children, whenever asked or even without being asked. "The world is our playground" is a wonderful sentiment. There is something incredibly refreshing about viewing the world as a place that provides the opportunities to be active, at any moment of any day, with the people that we care most about.

TIPS FOR PARENTS AND CAREGIVERS

1. Encourage your children to get together with friends to play actively outdoors.
2. Make time for outdoor family activities.
3. Model the behavior you want to see in your children.

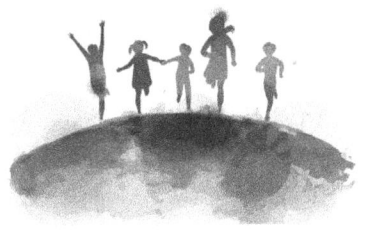

CHAPTER 9

Fun

Innovative Initiatives Helping Children Move More - Fun and Games as a Catalyst

D R. WILLIAM BIRD is a General Practitioner and the CEO and Founder of Intelligent Health. He created Beat the Street, which is a six-week program that turns entire communities into an active game. People receive maps and fobs or cards that they tap on "Beat Boxes" (contactless card readers) located around the city and surrounding areas. When tapped, the "Beat Boxes" light up and make noises. Points are awarded for each tap, which add up and can be redeemed for prizes such as tickets to sporting events or sports camp registrations. This encourages community members to use active travel to get to and from work and school, and to explore local parks and green spaces. According to one child participant, "it made me excited to bleep the boxes and made me walk or cycle further to reach them."[76]

Turning entire communities into an active game requires community-wide engagement. Engagement coordinators begin working with schools, workplaces, and other community partners early on in the process. Schools serve as distribution points for maps and fobs or cards and mobilize their entire student bodies, creating initial excitement and interest. Publicity events and social media campaigns throughout the game maintain the excitement and interest. During six weeks in the summer of 2021, a total of 60,187 people—or 11% of the entire population of the city of Sheffield in the United Kingdom—collectively walked, jogged, ran, cycled, scootered, and rolled a total of 452,870 miles.[77] Since it was first launched in 2013, Beat the Street has helped 1.67 million people get moving and improve their health.[78]

Dr. Bird attributes the success of Beat the Street to several key factors. The first is physical fobs that the children can touch and hold in their hands. The second is "Beat Boxes" that the children can see around the neighborhood. The third is leaderboards that add a competitive element between schools. The fourth is activities that the entire family can participate in, with children getting their parents, grandparents, and other relatives on board. He shares stories of parents who had never before been able to get their children to go outside to exercise being awakened at 6:00 am by them begging to go out to play Beat the Street.

Dr. Bird favors Beat the Street over how doctors typically approach the subject of exercise. Doctors liken physical activity to a pill and "prescribe it," for example, telling their patients to take the stairs instead of the elevator, or to get off the bus one stop earlier to walk home through the pouring rain. He criticizes this traditional approach as the opposite of fun. "Physical activity shouldn't be anything extra. It should be part of your well-being, it should be part of your life. It should give you the vibrancy and the additional fun in life. And if you can't do that then you are going to fail."[79]

According to Dr. Bird, there was a City Council member in France who was put in charge of the physical activity committee. The Council member decided to organize an event where community members were invited to use arts and crafts to decorate a local bridge. This inspired the city residents to walk to the bridge. He then did the same elsewhere, in parks and around waterways throughout the city. Again, city residents turned out to walk around these parks and waterways.

Dr. Bird reflects on this City Council member, who essentially created a catalyst. He stimulated people's interest and provided them a chance to see their surroundings and to realize that they could walk to these surroundings. Physical activity was the means and seeing the arts and crafts was the end. Dr. Bird notes that "physical activity should always be a means to the end… just a method of getting there."[80] If physical activity is the end goal, very few people will be motivated to participate.

During the COVID-19 pandemic, activity levels dropped as people sheltered at home. The most commonly cited reason for why adults were less active was concern about virus exposure.[81] In the UK, physical activity decreased 30% during the pandemic, and the largest decreases were among communities of color, the youngest and the oldest age groups, and unemployed adults.[82] As Dr. Bird puts it, "the divide got bigger"[83] in physical activity levels between different age groups and ethnicities, and the people most likely to be inactive got even more inactive.

Takeaways from Fun and Games Helping Children Move More

1. Fun, family, school, and community are elements that help create active communities.
2. Physical activity must be the means not the end goal in order to motivate people to participate.
3. Physical activity needs to be a fun part of life, instead of something extra.

How can parents and caregivers make movement a fun part of life?

Active travel is a great way to make physical activity a fun part of life, instead of something extra. Our lives are so busy that it is challenging to find time for daily activity, for ourselves and for our families. But every single day, our children need to get to and from school. Most days of the week, they also need to get to and from extracurricular activities. The easy choice is often to jump in the car for these trips. But the fun choice can be walking, jogging, running, cycling, scootering, or rolling to school and extracurricular activities. This is also the efficient choice as you carve out time for activity on your way to the desired destination.

Our home is about 1.5 miles from my daughters' school. Last year we used to drive them there after dropping their brother at his school, about 3.5 miles away. This year, they walk to school by themselves. Now, it is true that my daughters don't find walking in and of itself to be all that much fun. However, what they do find fun is walking to school with their friends. Every morning they arrange to meet up with one of their friends. They run to meet her if they are late, and they race off together once they meet up. They have so much fun with her on the way to school that they are eager to leave the house in the morning, so they are never late.

It is a win-win for us and our children. My husband and I save an hour of commute time, which we can use to do a walking meeting for work, and our children get the health benefits of walking three miles per day. They practice independence with the responsibility of getting themselves to school and reporting their safe arrival. They view active travel to school as a normal part of life. And they associate walking, jogging, and running— depending on the time and how close it is to the start of homeroom—with friends and fun.

How can parents and caregivers make movement a game?

Parents and caregivers can play active games with our children. Families were key to the success of Beat the Street. They joined together as teams. Children were motivated by fun and prizes and in turn, they motivated their parents and grandparents to be more active.

Parents and caregivers can also create the time and space for our children to play active games with their friends. My daughters have started playing an active game at school called "Groundies." Groundies takes place on a play structure, and it encourages climbing and jumping. The game participants decide who will be the tagger, and the tagger begins the game by counting to ten. The tagger can have their eyes open on the ground, but must have them closed when they are on the play structure. If they tag someone, they become it. If a participant hops off the play structure and they yell "Groundies" while they are still on the ground, they can also become it.

My daughters and their classmates are completely self-directed in their games of Groundies. They have so much fun that they play it all recess, and again after school. They love the game so much that they call or text every day to ask if they can stay later—and still later—to play "just one more game." I always answer "Yes" because I want them to keep choosing to spend time playing active games. I also want them to always associate movement with friends and fun.

TIPS FOR PARENTS AND CAREGIVERS

1. Encourage your children to walk, jog, run, cycle, scooter or roll to school and extracurricular activities with friends.

2. Play active games with your children.

3. Support your children in playing active games with their friends.

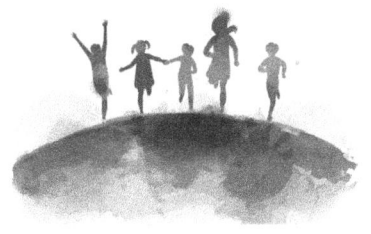

CHAPTER 10

Positivity

Innovative Initiatives Helping Children Move More - Feeling Amazing Through Movement

ZING! FOR KIDS brings physical activity programming to New York City schools and communities. Since March 2021, Zing! for Kids CEO and Founder Michele Levy and her instructors have been working on the frontlines of the youth mental health pandemic, the physical inactivity pandemic, and the COVID pandemic. Michele was inspired to launch Zing! for Kids because she recognized that schools were desperate for solutions, kids were desperate for a chance to move out from behind their screens, and parents and caregivers were desperate for activities for their kids.

Zing! for Kids starts every class with a "The Hype Up," which is a full-body warm-up accompanied by name games to break the ice and pep talks to get everyone motivated. Next is "Zing! Time," where kids do exercise circuits with intervals of cardio, upper body, lower body, and core exercise. After that is "Zing! Zone," combining team-based moves with stations and obstacle courses. "The Zinger" finisher is all about power moves and empowerment, and "The Cool Down" involves stretching and a motivational mantra. What makes Zing! for Kids different from circuit training for adults is the focus on play, fun, and positive affirmations.

A certified fitness instructor, personal trainer, and youth exercise specialist, Michele was not always an exercise enthusiast. In fact, she can relate to children who hate PE class, having been a very shy child who pretended to have exercise-induced asthma to get out of participating. Becoming a certified fitness instructor helped Michele break out of her shell and inspired her to help others become more sociable and outgoing through fitness.

Zing! for Kids is designed so that equal attention is given to children's physical health and well-being and mental health and well-being. The organization was born as youth mental health issues were coming to the forefront, and matured as children were feeling intense pressure to catch up in school. Empowerment is prioritized, as Zing! for Kids focuses on "teaching kids that movement is a way for them to feel strong and empowered."[84]

Positive affirmations are Zing! for Kids' secret sauce. Instructors make positive statements to kids, and encourage kids to say positive statements to themselves and out loud in unison as they go through the movements. For example, they can start warming up with lunges accompanied by an "I am smart and strong!" statement. They can move into jumping jacks that are accompanied by an "I am a rock star!" statement. They can cool down with the signature "I feel amazing, I am amazing!" statement.

Positive self-talk is related to higher self-esteem in children.[85] Kids feel stronger, braver, and more confident after engaging in positive self-talk. And the difference in how kids feel is visible to both themselves and the instructors. Their energy shifts when they hear positive affirmations from instructors, and then they start to talk to themselves positively, both out loud and internally. "We see kids really lighting up when they get to learn how to just move and feel okay."[86]

With Zing! for Kids Michele has created an environment for children that is the opposite of what she and her brothers experienced as children. Coaches and PE teachers didn't know how to work with them, other kids made fun of them for coming in last place, and they dreaded going to PE class. With Zing! for Kids, coaches act as mentors, cheerleaders, and friends—not drill sergeants. They create a safe space that allows children to come together to move their bodies freely while having fun.

Michele gets many of her programming ideas from calendars that track special occasions. For example, during National Superhero Week there are superhero-themed classes, costumes and moves that work on strength and agility. To Michele, success for this week and every week is seeing a child's face as they discover the joy of movement and their own inner superhero strength.

Takeaways from Feeling Amazing Through Movement

1. Movement can be a way for children to feel empowered.
2. Positive affirmations accompanying movement helps kids feel stronger, braver, and more confident.
3. Coaches act as cheerleaders, not drill sergeants.

How can parents and caregivers help our children feel amazing through movement?

Parents and caregivers can find a way to boost our children's confidence and self-esteem through movement. We can use positivity to associate movement not only with fun, but with strength and power. We can dissociate movement from pressure and worries. Somewhere along the line, as children grow into adults, exercise becomes a chore, something we "have" to do. What can we do as parents and caregivers to delay that as long as possible? Even better, what can we do to help them grow up to be adults who see movement as joyful, something we "get" to do?

Language is important. I appreciate and try to use positive language when I talk about movement. Not, we "have" to exercise but we "get" to move. It is a privilege that we get to move our bodies. We can use positivity in our own language, and encourage our children to use positivity in their language too.

When our children are worried or anxious in the face of pressures and challenges, we encourage them to use positive self-talk. They can say things like, "I got this!", "I am smart!", and "I am proud of myself!" We can also encourage them to use positive self-talk as they move their bodies. And we can make sure that the words that we as parents and caregivers use reinforce this positive inner dialogue. For example, if our children are saying "I am strong and powerful because I was able to run my fastest today," we can acknowledge and reinforce that statement.

Actions are important too. I am always so frustrated when I hear stories about PE teachers and coaches using movement as a punishment. "You were late, run five laps." Or "you lost the game, do twenty-five push-ups." Pairing positive affirmations with movement goes completely in the opposite direction from movement as punishment. Movement reinforces positivity and positivity reinforces movement.

How can parents and caregivers be cheerleaders for our children?

We can be cheerleaders for our children in so many different aspects of their lives. If they are nervous before a big presentation at school, we can remind them that they prepared well and that they always do such a great job speaking up in a loud clear voice, for example. We can also be cheerleaders about movement, whether we are tossing a ball back and forth with them one-on-one or playing a family game of touch football. For example, we can say things like, "good pass," "quick thinking," or "well played."

The scenario where we are most visibly and often called on to be a cheerleader for our children is when we are spectators along the sidelines during a match or a game. Although we have the best of intentions, parents and caregivers have moments when we can be anything but supportive.

I recently attended a soccer match where the father of a child on the opposing team hurled insults at his son throughout the entire game. There were constant critiques of the child's effort and his performance. I felt terrible for the kid, and even my son remarked on it after the game. It was distracting and uncomfortable for players and spectators.

I've noticed an increase in the number of signs directed at parents and caregivers on the sidelines of youth sports games, indicating that this is a widespread problem. For example, I've seen signs like, "Let the kids play. Let the refs ref. Let the coaches coach." Also, "The players are kids. The coaches are volunteers. The refs are human."

Critiques from the sidelines and in the car on the way home from the match or game are taking their toll. Kids become stressed and no longer feel like they are having fun. In fact, the number one reason kids quit sports is because it is no longer enjoyable.[87] Yet the number one reason parents want their kids to play sports is for them to have a good time. We have the best of intentions for our children, but the fun is getting lost along the way.

Although never to this degree, I know I am also guilty of being a coach and even a critic from the sidelines. I know this can impact how my children feel about the match or game, their performance, their team's performance, and even the sport itself. I have really tried to dial back my comments to three positive statements. "Nice ball." "Good job." "Keep it up."

I once received great advice from a former youth coach about how to interact with my children after a match or game. My immediate instinct is to dissect individual moves or moments of the match or game. Instead, I was advised to ask, "Did you have fun? I loved watching you play today. I had fun, too." I try to follow this advice every single time I greet my child after a match or game. It tends to be met with a smile, even after the toughest of games.

TIPS FOR PARENTS AND CAREGIVERS

1. Use positive language when talking to your children about movement.

2. Encourage them to use positive self-talk when moving their bodies.

3. Be their biggest cheerleader.

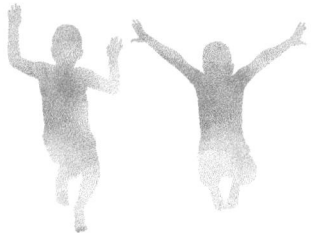

SECTION III

Academic Development

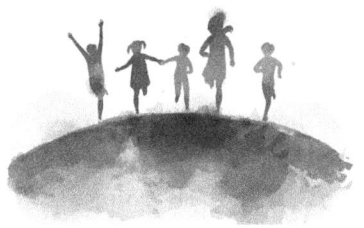

CHAPTER 11

Academic Development

ACADEMIC DEVELOPMENT IS the third of the three dimensions of Whole Child health that this book covers. What do we mean by academic development? Fundamentally, we mean learning. This includes the ability of kids to focus and concentrate, and to start a task and stay on task. We are also talking about progress toward educational and developmental goals, impacting performance in the classroom and performance on at-home projects and homework.

Teachers report that increasingly, students have difficulty paying attention. They are easily distracted. They have trouble regulating their emotions and behavior, which disrupts learning in the classroom.

This has a ripple effect in classrooms, as teachers spend increasing amounts of time helping students manage their emotions and behavior. With more time spent on classroom management, there is less time for teaching and learning.

The COVID-19 pandemic and widespread school closures were incredibly disruptive to kids' academic development. We could have foreseen that disrupting kids' education for months and even years would have a negative impact on their learning. However, we didn't anticipate the magnitude of the learning loss.

As part of the Education Opportunity Project, researchers at Harvard University and Stanford University developed a tool that allows people to identify the levels of learning loss in their local school district. Using this tool, we learned that kids in our school district in Somerville, Massachusetts lost, on average, 97% of a school years' worth of math learning and 43% of a school years' worth of reading learning.[88] The comparable numbers for the state of Massachusetts are 75% for math learning and 41% for reading learning. One reason the learning loss in Somerville, Massachusetts is higher may be due to the length of time our kids were not doing in person learning compared with other school districts. Our school district went virtual on March 12, 2020, and did not return to full-time in person learning until April 26, 2021.

To put this in context, student achievement among Massachusetts students—as measured by 4th and 8th grade math and reading tests—has now reached its lowest level since 2003.[89] Nationally, scores declined across the board, and the greatest declines were among students of color, low-income students, and English language learners.[90]

This learning loss has real-world implications for students that could last a lifetime. The math learning loss translates into a 1.6% decrease in the lifetime earnings of current Massachusetts students—equivalent to $23,840 per student.[91] Taken together, U.S. students could lose out on approximately $1 trillion in lifetime earnings.[92]

It's not just students who are suffering from this loss of learning. There are implications for teachers in the classroom right now as well. Teachers are feeling incredible pressure to catch students up. Schools are implementing a range of interventions targeting learning loss. For example, 30% of schools are spending more time on targeted subjects, 33% of schools have hired tutors to provide small group instruction, and 20% of schools have extended the school day.[93]

Despite these efforts, students are not catching up. National data revealed that half of U.S. students started the 2022-2023 school year below grade level in at least one subject.[94] This is the same as the 2021-2022 school year and 13 percentage points worse than a typical year prior to the pandemic.[95] At the current pace, third to eighth graders will need a minimum of three years to catch up, and some may not reach pre-pandemic levels of achievement before they exit the K–12 education system.[96]

As teachers try to teach more in less time, schools are becoming even more protective of classroom time. They are reducing the time spent on recess. For example, our school district has gone from two recesses during the pandemic to now having only one recess. Given that unstructured, outdoor, active play during recess allows children the ability to reset, refocus, and come back ready to learn, this feels like we are headed in the wrong direction. Physical activity is an additional intervention that schools can add to teachers' toolboxes to address pandemic learning loss.

Takeaways from academic development

1. Academic development refers to kids' ability to focus, concentrate, and learn.
2. Students lost six months to a year in math and reading learning as a result of the pandemic. They were still performing below grade level during the 2022-2023 school year.

3. Parents and caregivers can use the Education Opportunity Project tool to identify the amount of learning loss in their local school district, and use the information to advocate for interventions to address it, including physical activity.

How can physical activity help our kids' focus and concentration?

Kids who are physically active perform better at school. They have better school attendance, classroom behavior, and grades.[97] Kids who have higher levels of physical activity and physical fitness also have improved concentration, memory, executive function, and processing speed.[98]

Preschool children who are physically active have more cognitive school readiness. This is defined as the self-regulation, problem solving ability, and information processing required for learning in school. In fact, for every additional minute of moderate-to-vigorous physical activity preschool children did per day, their cognitive school readiness score increased by 0.20 units and their self-regulation score increased by 0.29%.[99] To put it in perspective, this self-regulation score increase is equivalent to vocabulary learning gains made in two days of pre-kindergarten.[100]

School-aged children ages 11-14 who participate in regular exercise during morning breaks have improved academic and cognitive function.[101] Using a sampling of children from this age range, a physical exercise intervention was conducted during the morning school break for a period of 30 minutes per day, 5 days per week, for 4 weeks. The intervention consisted of several stations for hand-arm coordination (e.g. throwing, juggling), strength exercises (e.g. circuits with burpees, lunges, sit-ups), balancing, jumps on stairs, and ball games. The students' reading skills, arithmetic competence, and attention and concentration ability were assessed at the beginning and the end of the 4 weeks. Results showed significant increases in attention and concentration, and in arithmetic competence.

How can parents and caregivers partner with schools to support physical activity?

Schools can increase students' physical activity before, during, and after school. They can support active transportation to and from school and provide programs, space, and equipment for physical activity before and after school. During the school day, they can provide PE, recess, and classroom activity breaks, as well as build physical activity skills.[102] The Comprehensive School Activity Program Guide for Schools provides step-by-step guidance to schools and school districts to help them develop, implement, and evaluate comprehensive school physical activity programs. The first steps include establishing a team or committee and identifying a physical activity leader. Subsequent steps include assessing existing physical activity opportunities, setting goals and desired outcomes, choosing the physical activities, and implementing and evaluating the programs.[103] Parents and caregivers can play a role in supporting Comprehensive School Activity Programs by volunteering to lead activities and encouraging principals and teachers to implement even more activities because of the clear linkage to academic development.

Dr. Rebecca Hasson is Director of the Childhood Disparities Research Laboratory at the University of Michigan. She focuses her research on kids, because she finds that reaching kids when physical activity habits are forming can be the most impactful. "And we can help to give them a passion and a lifestyle for moving more throughout the day that can hopefully carry into adolescence, young adulthood, middle age, and all the way until they are senior citizens."[104]

At this time, students need help with managing their emotions and behavior, and teachers need help with managing their classrooms. "All teachers recognize right now—after students were sitting at home for two years trying to learn successfully but in some cases unsuccessfully in a virtual environment—that students need help with their behavior management, managing their emotions, managing their behavior. And fortunately with exercise, almost any outcome you can think of, exercise, movement, physical activity can be a part of that solution."[105]

Recognizing that parents, teachers, and schools are overwhelmed right now, Dr. Hasson and her team have focused on integrating physical activity into classrooms rather than adding on new programs or activities. Some examples of physical activity breaks in the classroom include short bursts of activity, stretch breaks, marching or squatting in place, jump roping with an invisible jump rope, jumping jacks, and laps around the classroom. These can be combined with lessons, such as math with jumping jacks (e.g., $2 + 2 = 4$ jumping jacks) or geography lessons as children do laps around the classroom.

According to Dr. Hasson, active classrooms can take on many forms and her team helps teachers create a classroom conducive for physical activity. Specifically, "thinking about classroom management, thinking about the space, thinking about how to motivate their students so that they get the outcomes that they're looking for, so that the investment in activity is worth the time and you are… reaping the benefits of improved student behavior, improved focus, and attention. And eventually, as fitness improves, improved academic achievement."[106]

TIPS FOR PARENTS AND CAREGIVERS

1. Physical activity is an intervention that schools can add to teachers' toolboxes—along with intensive small group tutoring and extended school days—to address pandemic learning loss.

2. Parents and caregivers can encourage principals and teachers to take the steps outlined in the Comprehensive School Activity Program Guide for Schools to increase physical activity before, during, and after school.

3. Parents and caregivers can advocate for adding movement into learning in active classrooms. They can raise awareness about the large impact of physical activity on focus, concentration, and learning through short investments of time.

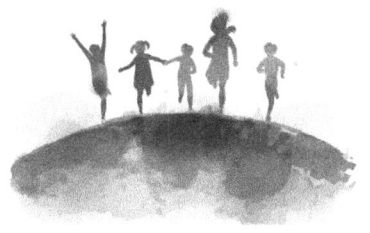

CHAPTER 12

Leadership

Innovative Initiatives Helping Children Move More - Learning Fitness and Leadership Skills

TARIK KITSON WAS volunteering at a school in East Harlem when he realized that many New York City school children do not have access to PE and fitness programs during school, after school, or on weekends. He had never thought about entering the nonprofit space, but was motivated by the differences in fitness offerings based on the geographic location of public schools. He found that the unfairness of offerings disproportionately impacted communities of color. According to a 2017 report, only one in five Black New York City public school students received the state-mandated minimum of PE class in grades K-5, compared with one in three white and Asian students and one in four Hispanic students.[107] Tarik found that public schools on the Upper East Side were able to offer a variety of in-school and out-of-school fitness programming—including PE, fencing, and skating. On the other hand, he noticed public schools in many Black communities were more likely to offer limited or no options, with the exception of basketball and football.

He disliked it when sports organizations came into a community and picked just a handful of promising athletes for their organization to sponsor. He wanted to start a preventive health organization that was inclusive of children at all levels and abilities. His vision was to work with all children—especially those who didn't really care about being an athlete—because he believes that all children have the right to know what it means to live a healthy lifestyle. According to Tarik, "you don't have to be a basketball player or a soccer player to be active. We want to be able to show kids the foundation and the importance of working out, of walking or running, how to do a proper push-up, how to run properly… this is important for you to just live a longer life, live a productive life, live a healthy life."[108]

He made his informal volunteer work more formal with the launch of his nonprofit, Active Plus, in 2015. Active Plus provides fitness, nutrition, mindfulness, and leadership programming to New York City's most at-risk children and teens. A New York City Department of Education vendor, Active Plus runs organized activities and instruction for dance, running, sports, nutrition, cooking, meditation, and yoga. In addition to teaching children about how to live a healthy lifestyle, Active Plus also teaches children about leadership skills and mental toughness, offers college and career exploration, and encourages positive self-esteem through its life and leadership programming.

One example of Active Plus's leadership programming is its Heal-the-Violence program. In 2021, Active Plus launched a pilot program in twenty New York City Housing Authority developments, in response to a significant increase in violence. The pilot program was funded through a city grant, and its purpose was to teach and model positive leadership. Youth and young adults learned tools and techniques they could use to de-escalate or prevent interactions from becoming violent. Following twelve sessions of "violence response" classes, community engagement discussions, yoga, meditation, and cooking classes, 78% of participants said they felt prepared to be leaders able to help reduce violence in their communities using the tools and techniques they acquired.[109]

Tarik noticed two distinct trends resulting from the COVID-19 pandemic. The first trend is that children who had their in-person education disrupted and who spent significant time at home became increasingly reliant on technology, and much less interested in being physically active. The second trend he observed is that schools are motivated to put more resources toward health and PE now, to address previous program cuts, because they see how dire the situation is. According to Tarik, "[W]e look at ourselves as emergency responders, because it's a state of emergency right now."[110]

Active Plus teaches school children, but it also teaches their families. Parents and caregivers join in for the nutrition and cooking classes, as well as the hiking and biking activities. A recent Citi Bike tour gave adults who hadn't ridden bikes since they were children the opportunity to tour from Washington Heights through Harlem and experience the joy and fun of riding as families through their community.

A quarter of Active Plus's program instructors are from the community and once participated in the program as middle school students. After graduating from high school, the previous program participants join Active Plus to teach these skills to the next generation of NYC school children. Those participants, in turn, teach it to their communities. "There is nothing better than being able to teach students and have them teach their colleagues, their brother, their sister, their family, other people within their community…"[111]

Takeaways from Learning Fitness and Leadership Skills

1. All children have the right to know what it means to live a healthy lifestyle.
2. PE and health education should include leadership programming in addition to the foundations of fitness.
3. Training students to be program instructors who teach their community members has a beneficial impact on the students and everyone in their communities.

How can parents and caregivers teach fitness and leadership skills?

Parents and caregivers don't need to be professional fitness instructors in order to teach our children foundational fitness skills. We can teach very basic movements, such as throwing a ball, jumping, and running. We can later progress to more complicated movements, such as throwing a ball at a greater distance, jumping rope, and running a relay race using a baton.

A train-the-trainer model of teaching fosters leadership skills at the same time that children learn fitness skills. For example, a child can learn a movement, practice the movement, and then teach it to siblings and other family members. This gives the child the opportunity to be "the leader" or "the expert." Being the most knowledgeable person in the room, able to share that knowledge with others, boosts the child's confidence.

Parents and caregivers can play games where our children take turns being the leader. Follow-the-leader is a classic. Every movement that the leader does can be a foundational fitness skill, as children demonstrate proper form for push-ups, lunges, and squats.

Teamwork fosters leadership skills, as children learn that they are working together to achieve a goal and that they have a role to play in encouraging their team members. Parents and caregivers can create opportunities for children to be active as a team, competing against the clock instead of against each other. For example, parents and kids can design an obstacle course together. Indoors, the obstacles can be pillows, chairs, tables, and stairs. Outdoors, the obstacles can be cones, bushes, benches, and fences. Team members high five when they complete a circuit, and compete against the clock, trying to improve their combined finish time each round.

How can parents and caregivers find opportunities for our children to practice fitness and leadership skills?

Youth sports provide many opportunities for children to practice fitness and leadership skills. The connection between sports and leadership is well documented. An often-cited statistic about women and leadership is that 94% of women in the C-suite (i.e., Chief Executive Officer, Chief Operating Officer, and Chief Financial Officer) played sports, including 52% who played at the collegiate level.[112] They credit their sports participation for developing the five winning attributes that made them successful as athletes. These attributes also make them successful as corporate leaders and entrepreneurs, and include confidence, single-mindedness, passion, leadership, and resilience.

My children rarely seek the spotlight in the classroom or on the field, although they are very capable when the spotlight shines on them. The difference is that they won't raise their hand to ask that it shine on them. Sports gives them the opportunity to take turns being in the spotlight, as the person who wears the captain's armband rotates to them or they make a particularly good pass that turns into the winning goal.

Children can practice fitness and leadership skills off the field and on the playground, too. After all, all children—not just athletes—have the right to know what it means to live a healthy lifestyle. Red light, green light is a great leadership game for the playground. Children can take turns being the person who stands at the finish line calling out "red light, green light" and judging who needs to return to the starting line. That person is the leader. When the leader says, "green light" and turns their back, the other participants move forward. When the leader says, "red light" and turns around to face the other participants, they must stop. If they are spotted making any movement, the leader determines that they need to return to the starting line. "Red light, green light" is already an active game, with walking and running involved, but it can also be turned into a game that practices foundational fitness skills. For example, children can dribble a soccer ball while moving forward on "green light," and trap the ball while standing still on "red light."

TIPS FOR PARENTS AND CAREGIVERS

1. Create opportunities for children to learn leadership skills while participating in sports or active play.

2. Teach children fitness skills so they in turn can be "the leader" and "the expert" who is able to teach others.

3. Play games that develop attributes that are characteristic of leaders, such as the ability to fail and try again and the determination to succeed.

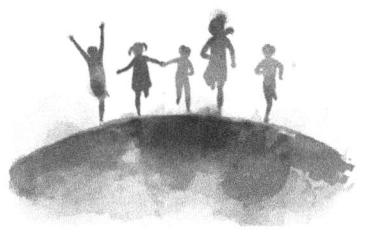

CHAPTER 13

Teamwork

Innovative Initiatives Helping Children Move More - Developing Teamwork Skills

WAYNE MOSS IS the Executive Director at the National Council of Youth Sports, an advocacy organization expanding access to youth sports. It focuses on the right of every young person to participate in sports in a safe, wholesome, and nurturing environment.

Wayne sees three levels of benefits coming from youth sports. For example, from a national interest perspective, sports help prepare young people to be fit to serve in the military and get people active early in life so they grow up to be active, healthy adults who are less likely to incur costs to the healthcare system. Youth sports also contribute to the building and investment in communities. Community is created as young people play organized sports after school and play recreational sports in backyards and neighborhood parks. On an individual level, kids gain physical, mental, social and emotional health benefits from youth sports.

According to Wayne, "We know that youth sports provide many benefits, including improved mental health and reduced risky behavior such as substance use, early sexual activity and delinquency. We collectively need to frame youth sports in that way so the public understands that this is not just fun and games."[113]

While it is important that youth sports be fun, they are not just about fun. They confer numerous additional mental and physical health benefits. And these benefits need to be communicated to the public and policymakers so that they take youth sports seriously and invest resources in them appropriately.

The National Council of Youth Sports believes that the skills learned in youth sports are critical building blocks for young people to become successful in life. In particular, Wayne emphasizes teamwork and leadership skills, as these are life skills that carry over into adulthood and "transfer over the course of a lifetime."[114] He also cites the Ernst & Young report that found 94% of women in the C-suite played sports.[115] He notes that a large majority of them attribute their success and rise to C-suite status to the lessons they learned from youth sports—including working as a team.

And yet, girls start dropping out of youth sports around age nine, because of lack of inclusive programming, lack of access, lack of role models, and gender bias. Wayne cites the statistic that by age 13, 70% of all youth have dropped out of youth sports, whether due to cost, poor coaching, overbearing parents, or lack of fun. To counteract this, he discourages parents and caregivers from coaching from the sidelines or after the game, dissecting what happened on the field. He encourages parents to instead "Let the coaches coach, let the players play, and let the parents cheer."[116]

The COVID-19 pandemic had a double-edged impact on youth sports, according to Wayne. On one hand, youth sports organizations that were operating on a shoestring, with small budgets and staff, ended up closing down for good. In fact, 44% of families said their community-based sports programs closed, merged with another program, or returned with a lower capacity limit due to COVID-19.[117] This disproportionately impacted the highest need communities.

On the other hand, there was a heightened awareness of the importance of youth sports. Youth sports organizations tried to keep kids playing sports outdoors, safely, when they had no other social or activity outlet. Moreover, there was a renaissance of recreational neighborhood play, as families and communities gathered safely outdoors to play sports.

Takeaways from Developing Teamwork Skills

1. The teamwork and leadership skills learned in youth sports are critical building blocks for young people to become successful in life.
2. Women executives attribute their success in part to the teamwork skills they learned in youth sports, yet girls disproportionately drop out of youth sports.
3. Youth sports should be fun, but provide much more than fun, including physical, mental, social and emotional health benefits.

How can parents and caregivers teach teamwork skills?

Organized team sports are an obvious place for children to learn teamwork skills. When my children were younger, they learned very basic teamwork skills like what it meant to be part of a group working for a common goal. As they grew older, they learned how to communicate with teammates and how, together, they were able to achieve more than they were able to achieve individually.

However, organized team sports are not a guaranteed place for children to learn teamwork skills. One season, my daughters played on a team where many of the players thought they were the only people who could get the ball up the field into the goal. They would try to barrel their way through a wall of opposing players instead of passing to teammates who were open on their right or left. They pointed fingers at other players when mistakes were made. They never trusted each other enough to pass the ball and have the confidence that their teammate would do what needed to be done with it. The coaches didn't seem to notice this lack of trust or spend time counteracting it by building teamwork skills and fostering a culture of trust. Thus, the children never graduated from a group working as individuals to a team working together.

Building teamwork skills needs to be an intentional part of both individual player and collective team development. According to national surveys on coaches and parents, parents significantly trust coaches to help their children develop life skills. Moreover, coaches of team sports value and prioritize helping athletes learn life skills above all else. In fact, the top three priorities for coaches of team sports are: 1) to help athletes learn new life skills; 2) to make sure athletes have fun; and 3) to teach the love of sport.[118]

Good coaches recognize how integral teamwork is to the success of the team, and they work to build teamwork skills both on and off the field. During practice, coaches prioritize, preach, and practice teamwork. They run drills that require the players to pass the ball a certain number of times before they can shoot, for example. Outside of practice, coaches organize team building activities like going to see a local collegiate or professional team play.

What can parents and caregivers do to teach teamwork skills besides signing our children up for youth sports that emphasize teamwork led by coaches who emphasize teamwork? Parents and caregivers can volunteer to serve as team parents for our children's sports teams. We can foster a team environment off the field by organizing team building activities like picnics, parties, and paintball. In addition, parents and caregivers can teach teamwork at home. Parents and caregivers can turn household chores into team activities. For example, we can set a timer and see how many toys our children can work together to pick up and put away in five minutes, or how many dishes our children can clear from the table together.

Parents and caregivers can also turn games into team activities. I became a huge fan of cooperative board games after I saw how uncomfortable one of my daughters became when we played competitive games. She would be reduced to tears by games like Sorry or Parcheesi—where players send other players back to the start in order to reach the finish first. Eventually, she opted to sit out of these types of games instead of playing. In cooperative board games, players work together to achieve a shared goal. They work as a team against a clock or a common opponent, never against each other.

In addition to board games, parents and caregivers can also play active games that teach teamwork skills. When I developed "Dr. B's Activity Hour," I included activities where children can work together to race against the clock instead of against each other. For example, children can run relay races where they try to complete a certain number of rounds in a certain number of minutes. They pass the baton or high five to cement the fact that they are working together as a team. They can even try to improve as a team by beating their previous time from round to round.

How can parents and caregivers find opportunities for our children to practice teamwork skills?

Parents and caregivers can play a very active role in finding opportunities for our children to practice teamwork skills. Signing them up for organized youth sports and turning household chores, board games, and active games into team building activities fall into this category.

In addition, parents and caregivers can create opportunities for our children to practice teamwork skills when they are with their classmates, friends, and peers. Parents and caregivers of younger children can actively lead games that foster teamwork at the park or playground.

For example, rock-paper-scissors in its traditional form is a one-on-one game with a clear winner and a clear loser. Two players count 1-2-3 "go." On "go," both players hold out a fist for rock, a flat hand for paper, or two fingers (index and middle finger) for scissors. Winning is based on a hierarchy—rock smashes scissors, scissors cut paper, and paper covers rock. The winner wins and the game is over for the loser.

Adding in a teamwork building component to rock-paper-scissors can turn the player who does not win the first round into the winner's cheerleader. They move on together to play another pair of players. Each round, the winner picks up another cheerleader until the final round, where there are two players and two teams cheering for one player or the other.

Children learn games at school during PE and recess. They bring these games with them to the park and playground. Parents and caregivers can encourage older children to spend time with friends at the park or playground. On their own, older children often have the freedom to make new and creative games based on old favorites. I am continually amazed by the teamwork focus of the active games my daughters make up together with their classmates. They describe scenarios where they help their teammates to safety, ensure their teammates all get turns, or free their teammates from imprisonment. They are collaborating, communicating, and reaching a shared goal together.

TIPS FOR PARENTS AND CAREGIVERS

1. Create opportunities for children to learn teamwork skills while participating in sports or active play.

2. Teach children teamwork skills on and off the field, as well as inside and outside the house.

3. Play games that develop teamwork skills instead of pitting players against each other.

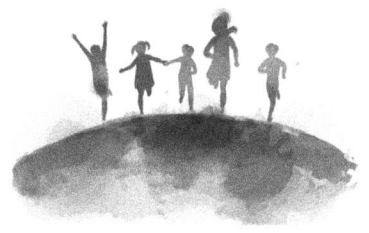

CHAPTER 14

Managing Risk

Innovative Initiatives Helping Children
Move More - Learning to Manage Risk
in Organized Play Environments

JILL VIALET FOUNDED Playworks—a nonprofit organization which has helped over 2 million students nationwide experience safe and healthy play every day—in response to an elementary school principal's plea to fix recess. She also founded it in honor of all the people who made it possible for her to play, and who helped her recognize the power of being outside playing and "mindfully in her body"[119] over the years.

Playworks involves coaches working with or training school staff and students to build inclusive play into recess. It organizes the play space and creates a shared set of expectations for the children at recess to increase their safety and ability to navigate the playground experience, as well as providing coaches and offering game ideas—both new games and variations on traditional playground games. However, the goal is to have the children and not the adults own the recess experience. Playworks does that by empowering the children, encouraging problem solving and turn taking, and developing leaders in the schoolyard—both informally and formally through the Playworks Junior Coach leadership program.

Jill sees play as involving inherently risky behavior, and notes that is a good thing. Children cannot learn how to manage risk without taking risks. Without play, children don't learn how to expand their comfort zones and "deal with…dangers and the metaphorical tigers and bears that are out there in the world."[120]

Learning how to mitigate and manage risk is an important theme for Playworks. According to Jill, "…ultimately, what you're trying to do is set these kids up to succeed. Not to eliminate risk, but to help them learn how to manage and mitigate and navigate risk in a way that helps them to be able to just thrive."[121]

Takeaways from Learning to Manage Risk in Organized Play Environments

1. Play involves inherently risky behavior, which helps children learn how to expand their comfort zones.
2. Children who learn how to mitigate and manage risk through active play are set up to succeed and thrive later in life.
3. Children can practice problem solving, turn taking, and leadership in organized play environments.

How can parents and caregivers help children learn to manage risk in organized play environments?

Risky play exposes children to stimuli that they may have previously feared while providing them with positive emotions. It involves challenging and adventurous physical activity they may have never done before. It generally takes place outdoors in both natural and built environments such as playgrounds. The benefits of risky play include helping children overcome their fears, reduce anxiety, gain self-confidence, test their limits, and develop independence. There are six categories of risky play: 1) Rapid speeds; 2) Dangerous tools; 3) Dangerous elements; 4) Rough and tumble; 5) Great heights; and 6) Disappear or get lost.[122]

Parents and caregivers can help children learn to manage risk in controlled play environments by addressing each of these categories:

1. High speeds. The risk is uncontrolled speed that can lead to a collision with something or someone. Examples include riding down a hill on something with wheels or sliding down a slide. Learning to manage the risk helps children overcome fears of high speeds or being out of control.
2. Dangerous tools. The risk is the danger of injury or wounds. Examples include using saws to cut wood or knives to cut food. Learning to manage the risk helps children feel trusted and in control.
3. Dangerous elements. The risk is the danger of falling into or from something. Examples include climbing on rocks or swimming in deep water. Learning to manage the risk helps children overcome fears of falling into water that is over their head or from steep cliffs.
4. Rough and tumble. The risk is that children can harm each other. Examples include wrestling or play-fighting. Learning to manage the risk helps children gain confidence in their physical strength.
5. Great heights. The risk is the danger of injury from falling. Examples include climbing to the top of a play structure or swinging from great heights. Learning to manage the risk helps children overcome fear of being high off the ground

and gain confidence in their arm and leg strength to get them up there or swing while they are there.
6. Disappear or get lost. The risk is the danger of getting lost alone or disappearing from adult supervision. Examples include playing hide-and-seek or going exploring alone. Learning to manage the risk helps children overcome fears of being separated, or not being able to find someone.

How can parents and caregivers find opportunities for our children to practice managing risk in controlled play environments?

Due to concerns about injury and litigation, playground equipment in the United States has become increasingly focused on safety. Think of shorter equipment with enclosed platforms, and rubber surfaces. However, decreasing risk has not translated into fewer injuries. Children have found ways to make less challenging playground equipment more interesting by, for example, running up slides or jumping off platforms and support structures. Even with the lower risk playground designs, there are about 200,000 playground-related injuries treated in emergency departments in the United States each year.[123]

In contrast with the United States, a number of countries—including Australia, Canada, Germany, Sweden, and the United Kingdom—are including obstacles and elements of risk as intentional features of their playground design. A sign at a London playground informs parents that risks have been "intentionally provided, so that your child can develop an appreciation of risk in a controlled play environment rather than taking similar risks in an uncontrolled and unregulated wider world."[124] Citing a 2004 Kambas et al. study[125] that showed children who improved their motor coordination in playgrounds at an early age were less likely to have accidents due to motor deficiencies as they got older, and with the backing of insurance companies that want to build "risk competence," these countries are adding risk back into playgrounds.[126] Their rationale is that people cannot learn how to manage risk unless they take risks, and children who learn how to navigate risk develop resilience and grit.

I am a risk-averse person with a risk-averse husband and three risk-averse children. It is hard-wired in our personalities. I have to remind myself to encourage my children to put themselves in situations where they test and expand their comfort zones. When they were young children, it was letting them walk or run without me holding their hands. Now that they are older, it is encouraging them to try new and unfamiliar things. It ultimately means giving them the freedom to go through life unsupervised.

The COVID-19 pandemic took its toll, making it even more difficult for parents and caregivers to give our children freedom to test and expand their comfort zones. Children and their parents had very real fears about what infection with the virus might mean for their health and their families' health. School and out-of-school interactions with peers and family members ground to a halt. Playgrounds were roped off, playdates discouraged. At times, it felt impossible to let our children do the things they were used to doing, let alone allow them to try new things.

The Let Grow Project—first brought to my attention by Jill Vialet—gives children an assignment. The assignment is to do something on their own that they have never done before, with their parents' permission.[127] Children are encouraged to identify an activity they would like to do that falls into the risky category. It might be something they are not currently allowed by their parents and caregivers to do. Possibilities include climbing a tall tree in the front yard, riding their bike to the store, or using a knife to make a meal. They come up with a plan and a proposal that they bring to their families, then they negotiate how they might be allowed to do that activity. After the negotiation and parental sign off, the children do the activity and report back to their parents and caregivers.

The Let Grow Project reports increased self-awareness, self-confidence, and reduced anxiety among children, as well as better relationships between children and parents. The experience is appreciated by kids but revelatory to parents. According to Jill Vialet, parental response has been extremely positive. For example, one parent reported, "that was really intense and amazing and made me recognize the extent to which I underestimate my own kid's ability. And I'm operating often from a place of fear. And that gets in the way of love."[128]

> **TIPS FOR PARENTS AND CAREGIVERS**
>
> 1. Find organized play environments for your children to safely experiment with high speeds, dangerous tools, dangerous elements, rough and tumble, great heights, and disappearing or getting lost.
>
> 2. Give your children the freedom to spend unstructured, unsupervised time outdoors.
>
> 3. Encourage children to identify activities they are not allowed to do but would like to do, then work with them to put a plan in place where they can test and expand their comfort zones.

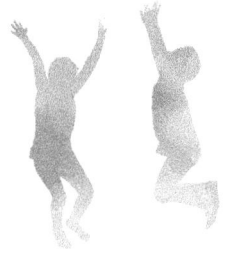

SECTION IV

The Role of Parents and Caregivers

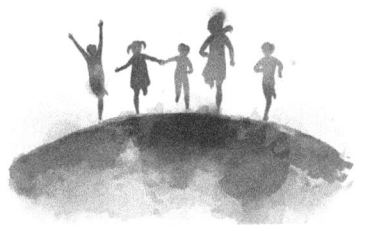

CHAPTER 15

The Role of Parents and Caregivers

THE PURPOSE OF this section is to explore the important role that parents and caregivers play in getting and keeping our kids moving. We can serve as role models, and inspire our kids to be physically active by demonstrating how we ourselves are physically active. We can talk positively about physical activity, and emphasize that activity rewards us with better mental and physical health. We can play actively on the playground with our younger kids and play sports and active games with our older kids. We can encourage our kids to be active directly, by giving activity-promoting gifts (e.g., sport and fitness equipment) and taking them on outings to places where they can be physically active. We can also encourage our kids indirectly, by setting up active playdates for our younger kids and suggesting that our older kids put down their devices and bike over to a friend's house.

There are several different styles of parenting. Psychologist Diane Baumrind coined three styles: authoritative, authoritarian, and permissive.[129] Authoritative parenting refers to high responsiveness and high demandingness, authoritarian parenting refers to low responsiveness and high demandingness, and permissive parenting refers to high responsiveness and low demandingness. A fourth parenting style, referred to as uninvolved (e.g., low responsiveness, low demandingness), was added by researchers Maccoby and Martin.[130] Additional parenting styles include various types of hyper-parenting, such as "little emperor" hyper-parenting (i.e., giving kids all the material goods they desire), "tiger mom" hyper-parenting (i.e., accepting nothing less than exceptional achievement from kids), and "concerted cultivation" hyper-parenting (i.e., scheduling kids into multiple extracurricular activities to provide them with an advantage).[131]

Parenting styles do influence kids' physical activity levels. For example, permissive parenting is associated with the highest number of minutes spent doing physical activity among children, while uninvolved parenting is associated with children spending the lowest number of minutes being physically active.[132] In addition, hyper-parenting is associated with lower levels of physical activity among children.[133]

In addition, parenting practices influence kids' physical activity levels. Parenting practices are the behavioral strategies that parents use to socialize their children.[134] Children who have lots of parental support—both logistical (e.g., rides to practices and games) and emotional—tend to be more physically active. Children who have highly protective parents (and therefore less independence and mobility), as well as lots of homework and extracurricular activities, tend to be less physically active.

The purpose of this section is NOT to point fingers at parents and caregivers. There is enough blame and finger pointing at parents

THE ROLE OF PARENTS AND CAREGIVERS

and caregivers already. Moreover, as parents and caregivers we do enough blaming and finger pointing at ourselves. Much of it is our own feelings of guilt and our own self-recriminations. *I should make my kids go outside more. I should have signed my kids up for basketball this season. I should spend more time playing with my kids.* We can drive ourselves to distraction with these kinds of thoughts.

It's also not my intention to place the responsibility of getting and keeping our kids moving solely on the shoulders of parents and caregivers. We do have some influence over our kids' activity levels, especially when our kids are younger, but this wanes as our kids get older. In fact, a systematic review of 14 studies looking at factors influencing physical activity participation in school-aged children found that the influence of friends ranked above parental influence as the most frequently mentioned interpersonal factor influencing physical activity.[135] A systematic review of 23 studies examining the means by which friends influence physical activity in adolescents found a positive association between physical activity participation and peer support, presence of peers in activities, peer norms, friendship quality, peer acceptance, and peer crowd affiliation.[136]

Parents and caregivers can most influence our children's physical activity levels during the time we spend with our children and the time we structure for our children:

<u>Before school</u>: Parents and caregivers can encourage our children to walk, bike, scooter, or roll (for wheelchair users) to school.

<u>During school</u>: Parents and caregivers can join together to collectively advocate for recess, PE, and active classrooms in our children's schools.

<u>After school/evenings</u>: Parents and caregivers can encourage our children to walk, bike, scooter, or roll (for wheelchair users) home

from school. We can sign our children up for organized sports or active classes, and help get them there and back. We can join together with other parents to advocate for active after-school programming. We can help our children find safe places to play and urge them to put down their devices and go outside to play.

Weekends/vacations: Parents and caregivers can plan active outings. We can get our kids to organized sports games and cheer them on from the sidelines. Parents and caregivers can try not to overschedule our children's weekends and vacations, and allow them time and space for unscheduled meet-ups with friends in neighborhood parks or on neighborhood playing fields.

Takeaways from the role of parents and caregivers

1. Parents and caregivers influence our children's physical activity levels, through role modeling, parenting styles, and parenting practices.
2. Friends have influence too, especially into adolescence. They are the most mentioned interpersonal factor influencing physical activity participation by school-age children.
3. Parents and caregivers can most influence our children's physical activity levels during the time we spend with our children and the time we structure for our children.

How can parents and caregivers make our children's environments safe for physical activity?

One afternoon while I was writing a chapter of this book, I received a call from one of my daughters. She and her sister had stayed after

THE ROLE OF PARENTS AND CAREGIVERS

school to play on the playground with their friends. Their active games are lively and complicated, and can go on for hours, so I wasn't expecting her call that early. When I picked up the phone, she told me their friend had been hit by a car while running across the street, chasing another friend as part of the game. There were nearby parents who were able to get their friend the medical attention she needed, but it was a terrifying experience for the kids and parents alike. Following the accident, my husband and I made a few adjustments to our rules, including asking our kids to keep their after-school games within the playground perimeter so they wouldn't be crossing any streets. We did not decide to restrict our kids' movement after the accident, though, because we recognize the incredible benefits of allowing them the ability to walk independently within our neighborhood.

Jeff Speck is a city planner who works to make cities more walkable and bikeable. He finds that for families to make the decision to walk rather than drive their car, the walk needs to be useful, safe, comfortable, and interesting. According to Jeff, safety is the category that needs the most attention because "most streets in America are designed in an almost criminally negligent way... encourag[ing] speeding well beyond the speed limits that are posted on the streets."[137] He cites, as evidence, that 82% more pedestrians are killed by cars in the United States today, compared with 14 years ago. He looks for ways to slow down traffic, asking questions such as, "Do any streets have more lanes than they need? Are any streets wider than they need to be? Are there adequate things like trees lining the street that cause people to slow down?"[138] He says, "Parallel parking actually causes people to slow down... When you remove the center line from the street, people go seven miles an hour slower."[139]

Parents and caregivers factor in safety when evaluating whether to let our children walk or bike to and from school, travel to and from neighborhood parks and playing fields, and play outdoors with friends. The Safe Routes to School program aims to improve safety and increase active transportation to and from school, and Vision Zero for Youth aims to eliminate traffic injuries and fatalities by improving safety in school zones and other places where children walk and bike.[140][141] Safe Routes to School programs were shown to increase walking and biking rates to and from school by 1.1 percentage point per year.[142] This is critical for counteracting the downward trends in the number of children walking and biking to school, which has declined by thirty percentage points over the past 50 years.[143]

How can parents and caregivers limit screen time and sedentary behavior?

The 2018 Physical Activity Guidelines urge Americans not only to "move more," but also to "sit less," recognizing the strong relationship between sitting time and health risks. They also note its high prevalence in the U.S. population, with U.S. children and adults spending approximately 7.7 hours per day (55% of their waking time) sitting.[144]

The American Academy of Pediatrics developed a policy statement on media use in school-aged children, which highlights media use as a risk factor for obesity. Accordingly, it recommends 2 hours or less of sedentary screen time daily. The American Academy of Pediatrics also recommends that families designate screen-free times and screen-free zones.[145]

Parents and caregivers can take several approaches to limiting our kids' screen time and sedentary behavior. One approach is to lead by example. We can model active behavior by choosing activities for ourselves that encourage movement over sitting. We can also suggest whole family activities that encourage movement over sitting.

Another approach is to make rules the entire family follows. For example, rules can include no devices at dinner or no devices in bedrooms. We can practice what we preach and keep our own devices away from the dinner table and out of the bedroom. The benefits will be better sleep, livelier mealtime discussions, consistency between our behavior and what we expect of our children, and, potentially, better work-life balance.

> **TIPS FOR PARENTS AND CAREGIVERS**
>
> 1. Learn more about how The Safe Routes to School and Vision Zero for Youth programs are impacting, or can impact, your community.
>
> 2. Establish limits on screen time.
>
> 3. Follow these limits on screen time and sedentary behavior yourself, instead modeling active behavior.

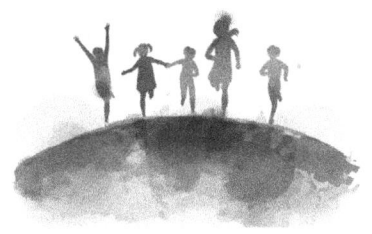

CHAPTER 16

Access

Innovative Initiatives Helping Children Move More - Expanding Opportunities for Children and Families to Be Active Outdoors

J**ACKIE OSTFELD IS** the Director of the Sierra Club's Outdoors for All Campaign and the Founder of the Outdoors Alliance for Kids (OAK). Formed in 2010, OAK is a group of 100 businesses and nonprofit organizations expanding equitable access to nature for children, youth, and families. According to Jackie, "we envision a just, equitable and sustainable future where all people benefit from a healthy, thriving planet and a direct connection to nature. And so, we're striving for a world where all people can breathe fresh air, drink clean water and safely and regularly spend time outdoors."[146]

Jackie is motivated by her work with children, and seeing firsthand the transformational power of time in nature. She has seen children with overweight and obesity who have built self-esteem and confidence through active time outdoors. She has seen light bulbs go off over kids' heads when they finally understand something that they learned in the classroom. She comments, "I've seen nature change us, I've seen nature heal us, and I just believe every child deserves to benefit from the outdoors, whether that's physically, emotionally, socially or academically."[147]

There are significant health benefits to being physically active, including improved brain health and weight management, strengthened muscles and bones, and reduced risk of disease. There are additional health benefits to being active outdoors in nature—whether it be an urban park or a remote forest. These include reduced stress, depression, and blood pressure, as well as increased mood, self-esteem, and well-being.[148]

Jackie is working to address the inequitable access to nature that exists for communities of color. People from these communities are more likely to suffer the consequences of environmental destruction such as air pollution and contaminated water. They are also more likely to suffer from asthma, obesity, and related chronic diseases. Yet, they are less likely—three times less likely—to have community level access to natural settings where they can improve their mental and physical health. In fact, Jackie notes, 28 million U.S. children do not live within a 10-minute walk of a park or green space. One of OAK's policy priorities is to ensure every U.S. child has safe access to public parks and open spaces within a half mile of their home.

Advocates are working to invest in transportation to increase access for underserved communities. They are also working to make access more affordable by reducing or eliminating park fees. The goal is to expand access for all children and families so that they can reap the health benefits of outdoor activity. Jackie sums up, "There is evidence…that kids, [and] families who have that neighborhood level access to green trees have better overall health outcomes, whether it's about obesity or mental health. But also, the mortality rates are lower when you have access to nature. And then there's evidence that suggests that all you really need to gain many of those health benefits is about 120 minutes a week."[149]

Takeaways from Expanding Opportunities for Children and Families to Be Active Outdoors

1. There are physical and mental health benefits as well as academic benefits to being active in nature.
2. Children can gain these benefits with just 120 minutes per week of outdoor activity.
3. Initiatives to invest in transportation and reduce park fees expand equitable and affordable access to nature.

How can parents and caregivers make sure our children get enough outdoor activity?

American families spend, on average, about 90% of our time indoors.[150] Most of the activities we have to do every day are done indoors, including sleeping, preparing and eating meals, housework, paid work, and homework. Similarly, most of the activities we choose to do in our leisure time are also done indoors.

When we are indoors, we are less likely to be active and more likely to do things while sitting, reclining, or lying down. Screen time—whether it's watching television, playing video games, or using electronic devices—takes up a lot (and increasing amounts) of kids' time. Nationally, four in five U.S. kids report engaging in more than two hours of screen time per day, earning us a D in sedentary behavior according to the 2022 U.S. Report Card on Physical Activity for Children and Youth.[151]

In contrast, spending time outdoors is associated with higher levels of physical activity.[152] When we are able to get our kids outdoors, they are more active. But getting them outdoors can be challenging. Part of the issue is a lack of infrastructure and safe places to play. Nationally, three in four U.S. kids ages six to seventeen live in a neighborhood with sidewalks or walking paths and parks or playgrounds, earning us a C in community and built environment in the 2022 U.S. Report Card on Physical Activity for Children and Youth.[153] However, only two in three U.S. kids ages six to seventeen live in safe environments, and there are large disparities based on race/ethnicity. For example, 72% of white children versus 57% of Black children and 56% of Hispanic children live in safe environments.[154]

As mentioned in the previous chapter as part of the discussion about walkability, concerns about safety—including traffic, violence, and strangers—impact parents' attitudes and actions and make us more likely to keep our children indoors or to drive them to and from places. Concerns about weather, such as extreme cold or extreme heat, may also play a role.

We can address some of our concerns about safety by spending time outdoors with our children, modeling and supporting outdoor activities. We can also foster independence in our children by encouraging them to go outdoors with their friends and stay safe as a group. We can address concerns about weather by adopting a resilient mindset and following the adage that "there is no such thing as bad weather, only bad clothing."

How can parents and caregivers take advantage of programs that support more outdoor activity for all children?

There are programs that seek to get U.S. families moving more outdoors. For example, Every Kid Outdoors, formerly Every Kid in a Park, provides free passes to fourth graders and their families.

ACCESS

The passes enable these children and their families to visit federally managed public lands, waters, and shores for free. They are good for the fourth-grade school year from September 1st to August 31st. Launched in 2015, the program reached 2 million children in its first two years. In 2019, Congress authorized funding for it through 2026.

In 1969, 50% of U.S. children walked or biked to school.[155] Today, only 11% of U.S. children walk or bike to school, and 62% do not walk or bike for travel at all during a typical week.[156][157] In 2005, the Safe Routes to School program was established by Congress. It aims to make it safe, convenient, and fun for children to walk and bicycle to and from school. Funds are used for the construction of bicycle lanes, pathways, and sidewalks, as well as education, promotion, and enforcement campaigns. The program has funded 14,000 schools in 50 states, raising the rate of walking and biking to school by 1.1 percentage points with each year of program participation.[158][159]

During the COVID-19 pandemic, my family noticed changes to many streets in our neighborhood. Signs were posted stating that they were "Shared Streets." The streets were open to certain vehicles, such as delivery trucks and residents, but gave pedestrians and bicyclists the right-of-way and allowed them enough space to use the streets while maintaining physical distancing. We used these "Shared Streets" constantly during our family walks after dinner. It wasn't just our neighborhood, though; a 13.2-mile network of "Shared Streets" extended throughout the city. Although started as a temporary measure during the pandemic, the state-wide program—which has awarded a total of $33 million to 183 municipalities to implement 310 projects—continues to fund projects improving transportation infrastructure today.[160]

TIPS FOR PARENTS AND CAREGIVERS

1. Model and support outdoor activity by spending time outdoors with your children.

2. Encourage your children to spend time outdoors with their friends.

3. Take advantage of free park passes and active transportation infrastructure that expands affordable, equitable access to outdoor activity.

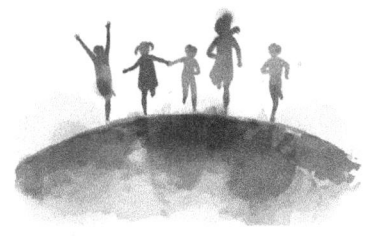

CHAPTER 17

Family Support

Innovative Initiatives Helping Children
Move More - Empowering Families
to Lead Healthier Lifestyles

TERESA EARLE IS the Co-Founder of the MEND Foundation. She is also a Co-Founder and Executive Director of the Healthy Weight Partnership, which was formed to bring MEND programs from the United Kingdom to the United States. MEND stands for Mind, Exercise, Nutrition…Do It! "Mind," represents behavior change and parenting strategies that help families make healthier lifestyle choices. "Exercise," is about families learning to enjoy being physically active. "Nutrition," is about families discovering that healthier foods can be delicious, nutritious, and affordable. "Do It!" involves motivating families to take sustainable action to lead healthier lifestyles for life.

MEND programs are intensive behavior change solutions focused on movement and healthy eating. The programs are usually delivered in community and clinical settings, including

YMCAs, community centers and Federally Qualified Health Centers (FQHCs). The core program is 10 weeks, with up to 2 years of maintenance and support. About 130,000 children and parents have participated in MEND programs in North America, Europe and Australia.

MEND's success has been attributed to the fact that its programs involve the entire family. It makes information accessible to children so they can process it and make decisions themselves about what they will eat and when they will exercise. According to Teresa, "We do it by helping the children become the agents of change in their families so that they gain the knowledge and the tools to help them live healthier forever."[161]

By working through the children, MEND empowers the whole family. The family unit benefits by having access to information on nutrition, physical activity, goals, and rewards. A family member accompanies the child during the program and thus, accompanies the child on their health and wellness journey. According to Teresa, "it is not a diet or a weight loss program, but health and wellness—a way of life for the entire family, for life."[162]

Teresa is motivated to do this work by the sheer scope of the problem—a third of U.S. children have overweight or obesity. She is also motivated by the fact that despite a weight management industry worth $59 billion, families still don't have solutions that are "easily accessible, affordable, personalized and, most importantly, effective."[163]

Demonstrating program effectiveness is another key ingredient of MEND's success. The programs are evidence-based and designed by child health and weight management specialists. Thirty-five peer-reviewed studies document the health outcomes of program participants, including reduced BMI and waist circumference, reduced sedentary behaviors, increased cardiovascular fitness, improved dietary intake, and better self-esteem and body image. MEND concludes it is the largest, most evaluated, and most effective healthy lifestyle program for families with children who have or are at risk of developing overweight or obesity.

Takeaways from Empowering Families to Lead Healthier Lifestyles

1. MEND makes information available and accessible to children, who serve as the agents of change for their families.
2. Together with their families, children use the information they receive about nutrition, exercise, and behavior to make informed decisions about movement and healthy eating.
3. The goal for program participants should be less about weight loss and more about health and wellness as a way of life for the family, for life.

How can parents and caregivers as a family unit learn to enjoy being physically active?

The first thing parents and caregivers can do is incorporate the spirit of MEND into our children's lives. As mentioned above, the "M" in MEND is for "Mind." It is about encouraging physical activity and nutrition behavior change. Long lasting, positive change starts with building children's self-esteem and sense of empowerment and supporting families with goal setting and positive reinforcement.

The "E" in MEND is for "Exercise," and stands for families learning to enjoy being physically active. For "Exercise," the MEND program's one-hour family sessions focus on such topics as being an active family, role modeling healthy behaviors, and physical activity options.

The "N" in MEND is for "Nutrition," and stands for families discovering that healthier foods can be delicious, nutritious, and affordable. For "Nutrition," the MEND program focuses on such topics as building a healthy meal, understanding fats and sugars, reading labels, and eating out.

The "D" in MEND is for "Do It!," and as I think about the program's focus on motivation and action, I think about three very concrete things parents and caregivers can do to enjoy being physically active together as a family unit. The first thing we can do is to travel actively to and from school together with our children. We can turn the trip to school into a race and the trip home from school into a game of walking backwards, for example. My daughters take it as a point of pride that they walk to and from school, no matter what the weather. They tell stories about arriving at school dripping wet but feeling invigorated from their trip, while their classmates have just rolled out of their warm cars and are barely yet awake.

The second thing parents and caregivers can do is to dance together with our children. During the pandemic, our family scheduled thirty-minute-long family dance parties that served as our activity and energy boost for the day. But the dancing doesn't need to last thirty minutes to have value. It can be for five minutes—a chance to get up off the couch during half-time or a commercial break. It can be for ten minutes—an opportunity to move and clean up the house together right before bedtime. All it requires is movement and music to make it fun, and all it takes is getting heart rates up to have health benefits.

The third thing parents and caregivers can do is to take an active break together with our children. When children sit for long periods of time, they lose focus. If they have a project due the next day and have been hard at work for a while, parents and caregivers can grab a ball and a glove and offer to play catch with them, for example. Active brain breaks give children a chance to reset and to come back to their homework ready to focus.

How can parents and caregivers as a family unit discover that healthier foods can be delicious, nutritious, and affordable?

As I continue to consider the MEND program's focus on motivation and action, I also consider what concrete things parents and caregivers can do to eat more healthfully as a family unit. First, parents and caregivers can plan meals together with our children. The kitchen is a natural place to talk about key principles for healthy eating, such as moderation, balance, and variation. It is a great way to teach children about the types of macronutrients, which include protein, carbohydrates, and fats. Parents and caregivers can help our children estimate daily servings for the food groups, which include fruit, vegetables, grains, dairy and meat/beans. When my daughter helps herself to one section of orange and tries to pass it off as her daily serving, we use it as a visual example to remind ourselves that one whole orange is a serving, and we need two servings per day.

The second thing that parents and caregivers can do is shop together with our children. This offers real world opportunities for parents and children to practice reading nutrition labels. My son is much faster than I am at figuring out math in his head. He can very quickly read, compute, and tell me, with a smile on his face, that he can in fact have ten servings of a certain food because it is still under the daily value for added sugars. Shopping together also offers real world opportunities for parents and children to learn the layout of grocery stores and how to comparison-shop based on price.

The third thing parents and caregivers can do is to cook together with our children. My daughters have gotten very interested in cooking during the past year. We started them out slowly, as assistants with meal preparation. They graduated to using sharper knives, and to cooking on the stovetop on their own. In just under a year, they have gone from being the sous chefs to the executive chefs, planning and cooking entire meals. It gives them a tremendous amount of autonomy in making meals that reflect moderation, balance, and variation, as well as building confidence in their ability to do so. As a bonus, it has expanded the universe of food they will try (and that they like) by a lot.

> **TIPS FOR PARENTS AND CAREGIVERS**
>
> 1. Work as a family unit and team, and practice movement and healthy eating together.
> 2. Actively engage your children in meal planning, shopping, and preparation, and creating and choosing physical activity options.
> 3. Make movement fill the gaps in your schedule, with spur-of-the-moment dance parties and active brain breaks.

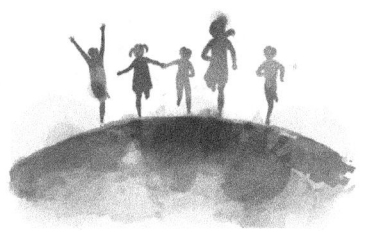

CHAPTER 18

Role Models

Innovative Initiatives Helping Children Move More - Modeling Active, Playful Behavior

PAT RUMBAUGH IS the Executive Director of Let's Play America. Let's Play America was founded in 2014 with a goal to increase opportunities for all people to enjoy play through locally inspired, playful events. She is affectionately known as "The Play Lady" for her work encouraging people of all ages to give themselves time to play daily.

Pat finds value for children in all different types of play—individual play, group play, physical play, and creative play. Much of the value of play comes from variety and choice, because, as Pat says, "not all children play the same. Some want to be alone. Some want to be with just one friend. Others want to gather and play in a soccer game. Some want to be very physical and climb that jungle gym, where others might want to sit down or go for a walk. It really varies."[164]

According to Pat, there are many benefits of play. For example, play is important for relieving stress. It makes us feel good about ourselves. It makes our bodies stronger. It gets us outside breathing fresh air. It gives us a chance to socialize. It encourages us to negotiate. And it teaches us how to listen.

Play is both a type of learning and a brain break from other types of learning. Pat believes that play needs to be recognized by school educators, administrators, and parents as being a benefit to—not a detractor from—academics.

But playing doesn't stop with children. Pat firmly believes it is important for parents to model the behavior they want to see in their children. For example, if play advocates want to see children playing, they should model playful behavior. Pat has a hopscotch on her driveway, open for business to all her neighbors. She enjoys watching people stop by to use it daily—kids, teenagers, even adults (who might look around and see who is watching before they try).

Pat built a playful community in Takoma Park, Maryland that, in 2010, was formalized as an organization called TakomaPlays! In 2015 it became part of Let's Play America. Takoma Park was also named a Playful City USA from 2009 to 2017. KABOOM!—a nonprofit that partners with communities to build kid-designed play spaces—ran this Playful City USA program. The program recognized cities and towns that ensured kids in their communities were getting the balanced and active play they needed to thrive.

Pat's dream is to build a network of play mentors. She has started to realize this dream by having older children serve as youth leaders at community events as part of their community service toward high school graduation. They emcee the events and lead games and activities. These older children model active, playful behavior for younger children in a circle of empowerment. "They are empowered by play and they empower others. They model play… when a child sees youth leaders, it makes a world of difference, because they're like, wow, if they can do it, maybe I can do it."[165]

Takeaways from Modeling Active, Playful Behavior

1. Children benefit from having variety in the types of play they engage in, and having the choice to play the way they like to play.
2. It is important for parents and caregivers to model the behavior we want to see in our children.
3. Older children can also be "play mentors" who model active, playful behavior for younger children.

How can parents and caregivers model active, playful behavior?

It is important for parents and caregivers to model the behavior we want to see in our children. We will have much more credibility and increased chances of having our children listen to us if we actually practice what we preach. If we are sitting on the couch working on our laptops for hours on end, while at the same time telling our children to unplug from their devices and go outside and move their bodies, there is a disconnect. It will be hard for them to take us seriously.

This is especially important for those of us who are parents and caregivers of tweens and teens. The odds are stacked against us if we want to counter the trend of children dropping out of organized sports by age thirteen, and spending most of their day on their devices in their tween and teen years. A 2021 study found that tweens and teens used screens for four hours and forty-four minutes and seven hours and twenty-two minutes respectively, per day, in 2019. By 2021, per day usage jumped to five hours and thirty-three minutes for tweens, and eight hours and thirty-nine minutes for teens. This was a faster increase in two years than in the prior four years.[166] If we are able to model active behavior for our tweens and teens and get them to unplug their devices and be more active, they in turn can model that behavior for younger children.

There are many ways for us to model active behavior by being active with our children as a family unit. We can play active games together indoors and outdoors. We can take family walks together. We can do fun runs together. We can play on the playground together.

There is also a place for us to model active behavior by being active away from our children. For example, we can join an adult sports league, sign up for dance classes, train for a race, or go to the gym.

As parents and caregivers, we often feel we can't take time away from our families to be active. Self-care is often seen as selfish, instead of a necessity to be able to be the best parent we can be for our children.

When we travel by airplane, we are instructed in the event of an emergency to put on our own oxygen masks before attempting to help those around us, including our children. I see taking the time to be active as an oxygen mask that helps me take care of my own mental and physical health needs. That way, I have the energy, bandwidth, and mental state needed to take care of my children.

In addition, it is important for our children to see that we are taking the time to prioritize our own physical and mental health. This will help them to make the connection between movement, and mental and physical health. In this way, hopefully, they will grow up to be adults who prioritize their own physical and mental health.

Prior to the COVID-19 pandemic, my family did spend time together being active as a family unit. However, generally, when I was doing activity for myself, I was doing it apart from my children. For example, I would go teach a strength training or cardio dance class at the nearby health and fitness center where I am a group exercise instructor.

During COVID-19 pandemic lockdowns, I did not have the ability to go to my health and fitness center to teach classes. I ended up buying a step and some weights and doing virtual classes in my living room. My kids would come in, watch for a bit, and eventually, they would join in—especially if it was a particularly fun class, like Zumba.

How can parents and caregivers model positive language about activity?

Using precise and correct language is really important when talking about activity. As a health communicator I spend a lot of time thinking about what language to use for which audiences. I think about communicating the health benefits of physical activity. I think about framing activity as fun rather than as punishment. And, relatedly, I think about framing activity as something that we "get" to do instead of something that we "have" to do.

It really bothers me when I hear stories about my children's PE instructors or coaches using exercise as punishment for losing a game, for example. To counteract that type of language, I try to talk about activity as a treat to be enjoyed. I also talk with my children about the health benefits of being active in ways that are relevant to them. I don't frame it as something that will help them prevent cardiovascular disease thirty years from now because a) they don't know what cardiovascular disease is; and b) they can't imagine themselves three years from now, let alone thirty years from now. We talk about stepping outside to reset, and we talk about active play as a way to feel less stressed.

Every Sunday, my daughter and I "get" to do a virtual yoga class in our living room. I inspire her because she sees it as something that is important to me, and because it is filmed in the studio where I teach group exercise classes. She inspires me because she is so motivated, and because her young and flexible body is able to do so much. She jumps from pose to pose while I creak in my middle-aged body doing those same poses. We have a wonderful time, and I think we are both grateful to have the opportunity to do this together.

> **TIPS FOR PARENTS AND CAREGIVERS**
>
> 1. Model active, playful behavior by being active with your children and doing activities that THEY enjoy.
>
> 2. Model active, playful behavior by being active away from your children and doing activities that YOU enjoy.
>
> 3. Model positive language about activity as a treat to be enjoyed, and something we "get" to do.

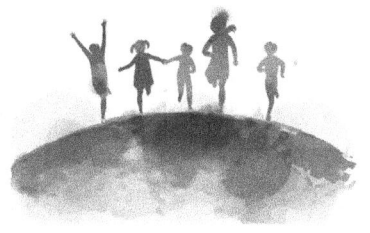

CHAPTER 19

Balance

Innovative Initiatives Helping Children Move More - Finding Balance

DR. JACQUELINE KERR was a public health professor and a behavior change health scientist who transitioned to being a podcast host and behavior change consultant. Her passion is helping people deal with burnout, particularly parental and working mom burnout.

Dr. Kerr's own experience with burnout forms the basis of her work. She helps companies prevent employee burnout and helps fellow parents avoid burning themselves out. It was on her own path back from burnout that she finally found herself in a place where she could "fix [herself], to do everything [she] could to become the better mom, the better boss, the better colleague, the better wife, the better friend."[167]

The COVID-19 pandemic shone a light on burnout. Teacher burnout was on the rise, with teachers retiring and leaving the profession, leading to staffing shortages. Worker burnout garnered media attention, with headlines about "quiet quitting" and the Great Resignation. Parental burnout became a serious problem, with parents trying to do their jobs while Zoom schooling our children, unable to find any semblance of balance.

Dr. Kerr attributes the high levels of parental burnout during the COVID-19 pandemic to a lack of control during very uncertain times. She also relates it to heightened levels of stress and anxiety as parents' work and home lives collided. In her words, "We couldn't hide the stress on the way to work or at work... And we were very much experiencing it in front of our children."[168]

Dr. Kerr encourages parents to be less judgmental of themselves, to recognize that they can't do it all well, all the time. She also encourages parents to reevaluate the standards and expectations that they put on themselves and that society puts on them. She cautions working moms in particular to not heap everything onto themselves and then to seethe and feel resentful that they have no balance.

According to Dr. Kerr, children watch how their parents adapt and cope with stressful situations. She reminds us about being the role models for our children that we want them to emulate. "We want them to see, you don't have to stand by the soccer field, you could go for a walk instead... we don't have to dedicate ourselves so selflessly to our work or to our children... having our own lives and looking after ourselves and prioritizing our needs, that's the life I want for my daughter."[169]

Takeaways from Finding Balance

1. Parental burnout became a serious problem during the COVID-10 pandemic. Parents and caregivers were unable to find any semblance of balance as their work and home lives collided.

2. Parents and caregivers need to stop holding themselves to impossibly high standards of doing it all well, all the time.
3. Children watch how their parents and caregivers adapt and cope to life changes and model balance.

How can parents and caregivers find balance?

As parents and caregivers, we hold ourselves to impossibly high standards, expecting that we will do it all well, all the time. Every day it feels like we do an entire shift working, and an entire shift being a parent, and it's almost like having two full-time jobs. The data backs us up. Parents today spend double the amount of time each day with their children than their parents did in the 1960s.[170] This is true despite the fact that more parents, and mothers in particular, are working outside the home.

Helicopter parenting, snowplow parenting, lawnmower parenting, bulldozer parenting, intensive parenting. These are all terms that describe a general trend of parents being over involved in our children's lives. This takes an enormous amount of time and energy, while causing us an extraordinary amount of anxiety and guilt. Moreover, it doesn't necessarily set our children up for success or happiness. If we are constantly removing obstacles from our children's paths, how will they ever learn how to overcome obstacles?

During the pandemic, this reached a fevered pitch. Our home lives and our work lives collided at the same time that we were expected to take on new roles for our children. We not only had to feed and clothe them, but we became their playmates as their contact with peers and classmates was limited. We also became their teachers, administering Zoom school and tutoring them in classwork and homework.

Parents today deeply appreciate just how hard it is to fulfill all their parental duties. 62% of parents say being a parent has been at least somewhat harder than they expected, with 26% saying it has been a lot harder. 41% of parents say being a parent is tiring and 29% say it is stressful all or most of the time.[171]

How do we feel less stress and pressure to be a perfect parent? We can't just snap our fingers and decide we are going to live a perfectly balanced life. However, we can make a conscious effort to prevent parental burnout by pacing ourselves. After all, parenting is a marathon not a sprint.

My children tell stories of classmates who shuttle from after-school activity to after-school activity. In fact, we hear many stories of overscheduled children who don't know what to do in their free time because they don't have any free time. Overscheduled children make for overscheduled parents, who race our children from activity to activity. However, recently, there has been a definite trend away from overscheduling children. Perhaps a silver-lining that emerged from the pandemic is that some families realized they preferred a less hectic schedule. My husband and I try to encourage our children to choose one activity per season as a way to have them prioritize their interests. It is a way for us to keep our family schedule manageable.

How do we judge ourselves (and our performance as parents and caregivers) less? We can't just declare our lives a judgment-free zone. However, we can remind ourselves that we are doing our best, and that's all we can do. Although parenting today is difficult, we do give ourselves credit for the good work we are doing. The majority of us rate the job we are doing as a parent as excellent (16%) or very good (48%).[172]

How can parents and caregivers model balance for our children?

Children quickly pick up on when we, as parents, are asking something of them that we are not doing ourselves. They are very quick to call us out if we, for example, lecture them on the evils of screen time despite being attached to our own phones. They also notice if we insist that they walk to school rain or shine but we skip our daily walk, using weather as an excuse.

Parents and caregivers can work on finding balance in our own lives, while modeling this balance for our children. For example, my children have to be at their soccer games at least thirty minutes, and sometimes sixty minutes, before kickoff time. Instead of standing around and watching them warm up, I try to take that time for myself. I usually find a hiking path (if I am lucky) or a parking lot (if I am not) and endeavor to walk the entire time. My children know that I am nearby if they need me and that I will show up before the referee blows their whistle at the start of the game. I recognize that they are not better off having me watch them warm up, but I am much better off for having gotten my daily walk in.

My children get very overwhelmed when they have large projects due for school. The idea of a project often becomes much larger than the project itself. A key skill set my kids are developing is chunking the project out into manageable tasks. They are then able to create a schedule that allows them to complete a task, take a break, then complete another task. More often than not, their breaks are active ones. For example, my son loves to play indoor basketball in his room.

As a small business owner, I view my company's operations as one large project, which is ensuring my company is successful. I am learning from my children how to chunk this large project out into manageable tasks so that I can complete a task, take a break, then complete another task. My favorite breaks are outdoor walks while I catch up on the phone with friends, combining much needed social connectedness and movement.

TIPS FOR PARENTS AND CAREGIVERS

1. Give yourself permission to not have perfection be your standard.

2. Encourage your children to pick one extracurricular activity per season as a way to keep your family schedule manageable.

3. Model breaks and boundaries for your children and encourage them to develop a schedule of manageable tasks.

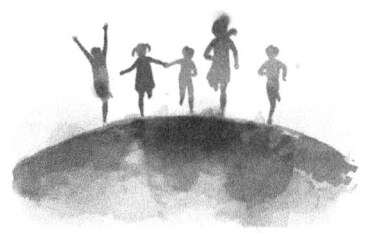

CHAPTER 20

Conclusion

PARENTS AND CAREGIVERS want what is best for our children. We want them to be able to successfully navigate the world without us. Above all, we want them to be healthy and happy.

But we see the data and the almost daily headlines. "The Kids Are *Still* Not Alright." And we see with our own eyes. Our children are not healthy and happy, they are depressed and anxious instead. They are behind in school. They feel cut off from their peers.

During the COVID-19 pandemic and in its aftermath, parents and caregivers have been on the front lines, witnessing our children struggling and feeling helpless about how to address it. I overhear parents and caregivers at the playground or on the sidelines, talking about which of their children had it worse during the pandemic. Was it their toddler, who had minimal social interaction and is now late speaking, or their kindergartener, who couldn't sit still during online school and is now late reading? Older children fared poorly, too. I overhear worries about a fifth grader, who is a year behind in math and feels so much pressure to catch up before middle school starts. Or a teenager, who struggles to socialize with classmates outside of school after a year of only seeing them in school. The worries and questions are endless.

I speak at conferences, where colleagues talk about the same problems at a much larger scale. We had hoped that children would be bouncing back in the aftermath of the COVID-19 pandemic. However, the news about the rising obesity levels, the falling physical activity levels, and the years of learning loss on national and global levels is dark and grim. One bright light, though, is this tool that we have in our toolbox—physical activity.

Physical activity is not going to solve all the problems that our children face. However, the linkage between physical activity and better physical health, mental health, and academic development is undeniable. If we could just get our kids moving more, maybe we could begin to tackle these problems that feel so insurmountable. It is a very concrete action step we can take as parents and caregivers for our families. It is a coping strategy that we can provide to our children, one with immediate mood-boosting impact.

My goal with this book was not to shame or guilt parents and caregivers for having children who sit too much and don't move. Rather, it provided a roadmap of 54 tips for parents and caregivers, containing words and the actions we can use to get our children moving more.

I have spent my whole career driven by my belief in the healing and preventive power of movement, and a recognition that every child has the right to experience the joy of moving their bodies. In this book, I shared what I do as a parent and caregiver with my own family to get all of us moving more. I shared what I do as a fitness professional to get my students moving more. I shared what I do as a local community advocate and the leader of a national physical

CONCLUSION

activity organization to change policies and systems to increase physical activity opportunities.

However, I understand that my perspective is only one person's perspective. Therefore, I also compiled stories about individuals and organizations that are making a difference in the lives of caregivers and children. They are helping parents and caregivers be active role models. They are helping children connect with coaches and teammates, as well as teachers and classmates, through regular movement. Their innovative initiatives focus on fun, fresh air, friends, freedom, play, joy, and games. They take place in homes, in schools, and in communities.

There are so many things that we can't control in our children's lives. That is one reason that we felt so helpless during the COVID-19 pandemic—our lack of control over our children's ability to have a "normal" childhood. This is true for physical activity, too. Although we can advocate for more PE, recess, and active classrooms, we have little control over the amount of physical activity our children get during the eight or more hours a day they spend in school and after school. We can advocate for playgrounds, green spaces, and sidewalks, but we have little direct control over the physical activity infrastructure.

There are, however, things that we can directly control around physical activity, including our actions and words. We can control the extent to which we model active, healthy behavior. We can put down our screens and ask them to put down theirs. We can talk to our children about the many health benefits of being physically active. We can sign our children up for town sports leagues. Then help get them to and from games. We can walk our children to and from school, and arrange for our older children to walk with friends.

This book is aimed to empower parents and caregivers to model and support physical activity, cheering our children on from the sidelines and playing tag with them on the playground. It's also aimed to empower parents and caregivers to monitor and discourage sedentary behavior, putting limits on our screen time and theirs to focus on active family time.

We as parents and caregivers have an awesome responsibility and opportunity to influence our children's ability, confidence, and desire to be physically active for life. We can teach them basic skills (ability). We can give them chances to be leaders on and off the playing field (confidence). We can support their motivation to be active in life (desire).

As we look ahead, we hope for a long and happy life for our children. We know that fit healthy children are more likely to grow up to be fit healthy adults with a lower risk of chronic disease. Move, to live longer.

But we can't stand by and wait for them to grow up to experience all the wonderful health benefits of movement. We need immediate solutions to help them with stress and sadness. Move, to live better.

My wish is that this book will both inspire you to get moving as a family and give you the tools you need to get started. Move, to live more.

Family dance party, anyone?

About the Author

Dr. Amy Bantham is the 2023 President of the Physical Activity Alliance, the nation's largest coalition of organizations dedicated to improving health and well-being through physical activity. She is also the CEO/Founder of Move to Live More, a research and consulting firm helping clients combine evidence-based research with practice for improved communications, policy, and strategy to get people moving so they can live healthier lives. A certified health and wellness coach, personal trainer, and group exercise instructor, Amy holds a Doctor of Public Health from the Harvard T.H. Chan School of Public Health. She lives in Somerville, Massachusetts with her husband and three children.

Endnotes

[1] "Whole School, Whole Community, Whole Child (WSCC)," Centers for Disease Control and Prevention, last modified February 9, 2023, https://www.cdc.gov/healthyschools/wscc/index.htm.

[2] "Whole School, Whole Community, Whole Child (WSCC)."

[3] "Constitution," World Health Organization, accessed February 23, 2023, https://www.who.int/about/governance/constitution.

[4] "Mental Health," World Health Organization, last modified July 8, 2022, https://www.who.int/news-room/facts-in-pictures/detail/mental-health.

[5] "Social Emotional Health," Kaiser Permanente, accessed February 23, 2023, https://thrivingschools.kaiserpermanente.org/mental-health/social-emotional-health.

[6] "What is the CASEL Framework," CASEL, accessed February 23, 2023, https://casel.org/fundamentals-of-sel/what-is-the-casel-framework.

[7] "Dietary Behaviors and Academic Grades," Centers for Disease Control and Prevention, last modified January 12, 2021, https://www.cdc.gov/healthyschools/health_and_academics/health_academics_dietary.htm.

[8] "Physical Activity and Sedentary Behaviors and Academic Grades," Centers for Disease Control and Prevention, last modified January 12, 2021, https://www.cdc.gov/healthyschools/health_and_academics/physical-activity-and-sedentary-behaviors-and-academic-grades.htm.

[9] "More Comprehensive State Guidance Can Support the Whole Child During COVID-19," Child Trends, last modified January 14, 2021, https://www.childtrends.org/publications/more-comprehensive-state-guidance-support-whole-child-covid-19.

[10] Rob Bisceglie, Podcast recording with author, October 18, 2022.

11 "Family School Partnerships," Action for Healthy Kids, accessed February 23, 2023, https://www.actionforhealthykids.org/learn-more-family-school-partnerships.

12 Rob Bisceglie, Podcast recording with author, October 18, 2022.

13 "Promoting Health for Children and Adolescents," Centers for Disease Control and Prevention, last modified May 23, 2022, https://www.cdc.gov/chronicdisease/resources/publications/factsheets/children-health.htm.

14 "Health Benefits of Physical Activity for Children, Centers for Disease Control and Prevention, last modified January 12, 2022, https://www.cdc.gov/physicalactivity/basics/adults/health-benefits-of-physical-activity-for-children.html.

15 Simon Kolb et al., "Indicators to Assess Physical Health of Children and Adolescents in Activity Research-A Scoping Review," *International Journal of Environmental Research and Public Health* 18, no. 20: 10711, https://doi.org/10.3390/ijerph182010711.

16 Risto Telama et al., "Physical Activity from Childhood to Adulthood: A 21-year Tracking Study" *American Journal of Preventive Medicine* 28, no. 3 (April 2005): 267-273 https://doi.org/10.1016/j.amepre.2004.12.003.

17 "NHANES 2017-March 2020 Pre-pandemic," Centers for Disease Control and Prevention, accessed March 2, 2023, https://wwwn.cdc.gov/nchs/nhanes/continuousnhanes/default.aspx?cycle=2017-2020.

18 Regina Guthold et al., "Global Trends in Insufficient Physical Activity Among Adolescents: A Pooled Analysis of 298 Population-based Surveys with 1.6 million Participants, *Lancet Child and Adolescent Health* 4, no. 1 (2020):23-35, https://doi.org/10.1016/s2352-4642(19)30323-2.

19 "National Survey of Children's Health Interactive Data," Data Resource Center for Child & Adolescent Health, accessed March 2, 2023, https://www.childhealthdata.org.

20 Ross D. Neville et al., "Global Changes in Child and Adolescent Physical Activity During the COVID-19 Pandemic: A Systematic Review and Meta-analysis," *JAMA Pediatrics* 176, no. 9 (2022): 886–894, https://doi.org/10.1001/jamapediatrics.2022.2313.

21 Genevieve F. Dunton, Bridgette Do, and Shirlene D. Wang, "Early Effects of the COVID-19 Pandemic on Physical Activity and Sedentary

Behavior in Children Living in the U.S.," *BMC Public Health* 20, no. 1351 (2020), https://doi.org/10.1186/s12889-020-09429-3.

[22] Carl J. Caspersen, Kenneth E. Powell, and Gregory M. Christenson, "Physical Activity, Exercise, and Physical Fitness: Definitions and Distinctions for Health-Related Research," *Public Health Reports* 100, no. 2 (March-April 1985): 126–131, https://pubmed.ncbi.nlm.nih.gov/3920711.

[23] Claude Bouchard and Roy J. Shephard, "Physical Activity, Fitness and Health : The Model and Key Concepts," in *Physical Activity, Fitness, and Health: International Proceedings and Consensus Statement,* eds. Claude Bouchard, Roy J. Shepherd, and Thomas Stephens (Human Kinetics Publishers, 1994), 77-88, https://psycnet.apa.org/record/1994-97580-003.

[24] Jaime Gahche et al., "Cardiorespiratory Fitness Levels Among U.S. Youth Aged 12-15 Years: United States, 1999-2004 and 2012," *NCHS Data Brief* no. 153 (May 2014): 1-8, https://pubmed.ncbi.nlm.nih.gov/24871993.

[25] "Childhood Obesity Facts," Centers for Disease Control and Prevention, last modified May 17, 2022, https://www.cdc.gov/obesity/data/childhood.html.

[26] "Childhood Obesity Facts."

[27] Samantha J. Lange et al., "Longitudinal Trends in Body Mass Index Before and During the COVID-19 Pandemic Among Persons Aged 2–19 Years — United States, 2018–2020," Morbidity and Mortality Weekly Report no. 70 (2021): 1278–1283, http://dx.doi.org/10.15585/mmwr.mm7037a3.

[28] Lange et al., "Longitudinal Trends."

[29] Mark Simmonds et al., "Predicting Adult Obesity from Childhood Obesity: A Systematic Review and Meta-Analysis." *Obesity Reviews* 17, no. 2 (December 23, 2015): 95–107. https://doi.org/10.1111/obr.12334.

[30] Sarah E. Hampl et al., "Clinical Practice Guideline for the Evaluation and Treatment of Children and Adolescents With Obesity." *Pediatrics* 151, no. 2 (January 9, 2023). https://doi.org/10.1542/peds.2022-060640.

[31] Catherine Pearson, "New Guidelines Underscore How Complicated Childhood Obesity Is for Patients and Providers," *New York Times*, January 20, 2023, https://www.nytimes.com/2023/01/20/well/family/childhood-obesity-guidelines.html.

32 "About Active People, Healthy Nation℠," Centers for Disease Control and Prevention, last modified June 3, 2022, https://www.cdc.gov/physicalactivity/activepeoplehealthynation/about-active-people-healthy-nation.html.

33 "About Active People, Healthy Nation℠."

34 Ken Rose, Podcast recording with author, July 26, 2022.

35 "Physical Activity Guidelines for School-Aged Children and Adolescents," Centers for Disease Control and Prevention, last modified July 26, 2022, https://www.cdc.gov/healthyschools/physicalactivity/guidelines.htm.

36 "Materials for Parents," U.S. Department of Health and Human Services, last modified May 25, 2023, https://health.gov/our-work/nutrition-physical-activity/move-your-way-community-resources/campaign-materials/materials-parents.

37 STOP Obesity Alliance and Alliance for a Healthier Generation, *Weigh In: Talking to Your Children About Weight and Health*, https://www.apa.org/obesity-guideline/discussing-weight/talking-to-children.pdf.

38 Ken Rose, Podcast recording with author, July 26, 2022.

39 Daniel Fulham O'Neill, Podcast recording with author, May 5, 2021.

40 Daniel Fulham O'Neill, Podcast recording with author, May 5, 2021.

41 Daniel Fulham O'Neill, Podcast recording with author, May 5, 2021.

42 Daniel Fulham O'Neill, Podcast recording with author, May 5, 2021.

43 Elaine Wyllie, Podcast recording with author, June 16, 2021.

44 Emily Marchant et al., "The Daily Mile: Whole-School Recommendations for Implementation and Sustainability. A Mixed-Methods Study." *PLOS ONE* 15, no. 2 (February 5, 2020): e0228149, https://doi.org/10.1371/journal.pone.0228149.

45 Elaine Wyllie, Podcast recording with author, June 16, 2021.

46 Elaine Wyllie, Podcast recording with author, June 16, 2021.

47 Josephine N. Booth, "A Citizen Science Study of Short Physical Activity Breaks at School: Improvements in Cognition and Wellbeing with Self-Paced Activity." *BMC Medicine* 18, no. 1 (March 17, 2020), https://doi.org/10.1186/s12916-020-01539-4.

48 Elaine Wyllie, Podcast recording with author, June 16, 2021.

ENDNOTES

[49] The Aspen Institute Project Play, *Physical Literacy in the United States: A Model, Strategic Plan, and Call to Action*, https://www.aspeninstitute.org/wp-content/uploads/2020/03/PhysicalLiteracy_ExecSum_AspenInstitute.pdf.

[50] Chuck Runyon, Podcast recording with author, June 14, 2020.

[51] Chuck Runyon, Podcast recording with author, June 14, 2020.

[52] Chuck Runyon, Podcast recording with author, June 14, 2020.

[53] Walter R. Thompson, "Worldwide Survey of Fitness Trends for 2023." *Acsm's Health & Fitness Journal* 27, no. 1 (January 1, 2023): 9–18, https://doi.org/10.1249/fit.0000000000000834.

[54] "What is Mental Health?," Substance Abuse and Mental Health Services Administration, last modified April 24, 2023, https://www.samhsa.gov/mental-health.

[55] "Health and Well-being," World Health Organization, accessed March 10, 2023, https://www.who.int/data/gho/data/major-themes/health-and-well-being.

[56] Nicole Racine et al., "Global Prevalence of Depressive and Anxiety Symptoms in Children and Adolescents During COVID-19: A Meta-analysis," *JAMA Pediatrics* 175, no.11 (2021):1142–1150, https://doi.org/10.1001/jamapediatrics.2021.2482.

[57] Valerie J. Calderon, "U.S. Parents Say COVID-19 Harming Child's Mental Health," Gallup, June 16, 2020, https://news.gallup.com/poll/312605/parents-say-covid-harming-child-mental-health.aspx.

[58] "National Survey: Youth Well-Being During COVID-19," The Jed Foundation, January 29, 2021, https://jedfoundation.org/national-survey-youth-well-being-during-covid-19.

[59] "National Survey: Youth Well-Being During COVID-19."

[60] "National Survey: Youth Well-Being During COVID-19."

[61] "AAP-AACAP-CHA Declaration of a National Emergency in Child and Adolescent Mental Health," American Academy of Pediatrics, last modified October 19, 2021, https://www.aap.org/en/advocacy/child-and-adolescent-healthy-mental-development/aap-aacap-cha-declaration-of-a-national-emergency-in-child-and-adolescent-mental-health.

[62] Office of the Surgeon General, *Protecting Youth Mental Health: The U.S. Surgeon General's Advisory*, Washington, DC: US Department of

Health and Human Services, 2021, https://www.hhs.gov/sites/default/files/surgeon-general-youth-mental-health-advisory.pdf.

[63] "Data and Statistics on Children's Mental Health," Centers for Disease Control and Prevention, last modified March 8, 2023, https://www.cdc.gov/childrensmentalhealth/data.html.

[64] "Data and Statistics on Children's Mental Health."

[65] Jean M. Twenge, "The Sad State of Happiness in the United States and the Role of Digital Media," *World Happiness Report 2019*, https://s3.amazonaws.com/happiness-report/2019/WHR19_Ch5.pdf.

[66] Twenge, "The Sad State of Happiness in the United States and the Role of Digital Media."

[67] David Axelson, "Beyond A Bigger Workforce: Addressing the Shortage of Child and Adolescent Psychiatrists," Pediatrics Nationwide, April 10, 2020, https://pediatricsnationwide.org/2020/04/10/beyond-a-bigger-workforce-addressing-the-shortage-of-child-and-adolescent-psychiatrists.

[68] Xihe Zhu, Justin A. Haegele, and Seán Healy, "Movement and Mental Health: Behavioral Correlates of Anxiety and Depression Among Children of 6–17 years old in the U.S.," *Mental Health and Physical Activity* 16 (March 2019): 60-65, https://doi.org/10.1016/j.mhpa.2019.04.002.

[69] Aaron Kandola et al., "Depressive Symptoms and Objectively Measured Physical Activity and Sedentary Behaviour throughout Adolescence: A Prospective Cohort Study," *The Lancet Psychiatry* 7, no. 3 (March 1, 2020): 262–71, https://doi.org/10.1016/s2215-0366(20)30034-1.

[70] Rachel Minkin and Juliana Menasce Horowitz, "Parenting in America Today," Pew Research Center, January 24, 2023, https://www.pewresearch.org/social-trends/2023/01/24/parenting-in-america-today.

[71] Brendon Stubbs, Podcast recording with author, June 30, 2021.

[72] "Data and Statistics on Children's Mental Health."

[73] Janet Omstead, Podcast recording with author, April 21, 2021.

[74] Janet Omstead, Podcast recording with author, April 21, 2021.

[75] Janet Omstead, Podcast recording with author, April 21, 2021.

ENDNOTES

76 "Beat the Street Sheffield 2021 Post Game Report," Move More Sheffield, https://www.movemoresheffield.com/beatthestreet.

77 "Beat the Street Sheffield 2021 Post Game Report."

78 "Beat the Street," Intelligent Health, accessed July 9, 2023, https://www.intelligenthealth.co.uk/programmes/beat-the-street.

79 William Bird, Podcast recording with author, August 31, 2021.

80 William Bird, Podcast recording with author, August 31, 2021.

81 Kathleen B. Watson et al., "Cross-Sectional Study of Changes in Physical Activity Behavior during the COVID-19 Pandemic among US Adults." *International Journal of Behavioral Nutrition and Physical Activity* 18, no. 1 (July 7, 2021), https://doi.org/10.1186/s12966-021-01161-4.

82 Tessa Strain, "Population Level Physical Activity before and during the First National COVID-19 Lockdown: A Nationally Representative Repeat Cross-Sectional Study of 5 Years of Active Lives Data in England." *The Lancet Regional Health* 12 (January 1, 2022): 100265, https://doi.org/10.1016/j.lanepe.2021.100265.

83 William Bird, Podcast recording with author, August 31, 2021.

84 Michele Levy, Podcast recording with author, June 28, 2022.

85 Paul C. Burnett, "Self-Talk in Upper Elementary School Children: Its Relationship with Irrational Beliefs, Self-Esteem, and Depression." *Journal of Rational-Emotive & Cognitive-Behavior Therapy* 12, no. 3 (September 1, 1994): 181–88, https://doi.org/10.1007/bf02354595.

86 Michele Levy, Podcast recording with author, June 28, 2022.

87 Jon Solomon, "Survey: Kids Quit Most Sports by Age 11," Aspen Institute Project Play, August 1, 2019, https://projectplay.org/news/kids-quit-most-sports-by-age-11.

88 "2019-2022 Change in Average Math Scores; 2019-2022 Change in Average Reading Scores," Education Opportunity Project at Stanford University, accessed March 20, 2023, https://edopportunity.org/recovery.

89 "The Nation's Report Card," National Assessment of Educational Progress, accessed March 20, 2023, https://nces.ed.gov/nationsreportcard.

90 "The Nation's Report Card."

[91] Thomas J. Kane et al., *What Do Changes in State Test Scores Imply for Later Life Outcomes?*, Cambridge, MA: Center for Education Policy Research, Harvard University, October 2022, https://educationrecoveryscorecard.org/wp-content/uploads/2022/10/Long-Term-Outcomes.pdf.

[92] Kane et al., ""What Do Changes in State Test Scores Imply for Later Life Outcomes?"

[93] National Center for Education Statistics, accessed March 20, 2023, https://nces.ed.gov.

[94] National Center for Education Statistics, accessed March 20, 2023, https://nces.ed.gov.

[95] National Center for Education Statistics, accessed March 20, 2023, https://nces.ed.gov.

[96] Maria V. Carbonari et al., *The Challenges of Implementing Academic COVID Recovery Interventions: Evidence from The Road to Recovery Project*, CALDER Working Paper No. 275-1122, November 2022, https://caldercenter.org/sites/default/files/CALDER%20WP%20275-1222.pdf.

[97] "Physical Activity Facts," Centers for Disease Control and Prevention, last modified July 26, 2022, https://www.cdc.gov/healthyschools/physicalactivity/facts.htm.

[98] "Physical Activity Facts."

[99] Pulan Bai et al., "The Relationship between Physical Activity, Self-Regulation and Cognitive School Readiness in Preschool Children," *International Journal of Environmental Research and Public Health* 18, no. 22 (November 10, 2021): 11797, https://doi.org/10.3390/ijerph182211797.

[100] Megan M. McClelland et al., "Links between Behavioral Regulation and Preschoolers' Literacy, Vocabulary, and Math Skills," *Developmental Psychology* 43, no. 4 (January 1, 2007): 947–59. https://doi.org/10.1037/0012-1649.43.4.947.

[101] Markus Tilp, "Physical Exercise During the Morning School-Break Improves Basic Cognitive Functions," *Mind, Brain, and Education* 14, no. 1 (November 26, 2019): 24–31, https://doi.org/10.1111/mbe.12228.

[102] Physical Activity Guidelines for Americans Midcourse Report Subcommittee of the President's Council on Fitness, Sports &

ENDNOTES

Nutrition, *Physical Activity Guidelines for Americans Midcourse Report: Strategies to Increase Physical Activity Among Youth*, Washington, DC: U.S. Department of Health and Human Services, 2012, https://health.gov/sites/default/files/2019-09/pag-mid-course-report-final.pdf.

[103] Centers for Disease Control and Prevention, *Comprehensive School Physical Activity Programs: A Guide for Schools*, Atlanta, GA: U.S. Department of Health and Human Services, 2013, https://www.cdc.gov/healthyschools/ physicalactivity/pdf/13_242620-A_CSPAP_SchoolPhysActivityPrograms_Final_508_12192013.pdf.

[104] Rebecca Hasson, Podcast recording with author, February 7, 2023.

[105] Rebecca Hasson, Podcast recording with author, February 7, 2023.

[106] Rebecca Hasson, Podcast recording with author, February 7, 2023.

[107] New York Lawyers for the Public Interest, *Leveling the Playing Field: Access to Physical Education in New York City's Public School System*, June 2017, https://nylpi.org/wp-content/uploads/2017/07/Leveling_playing_field_v11.pdf.

[108] Tarik Kitson, Podcast recording with author, September 6, 2022.

[109] Active Plus, *2021 Annual Report*, https://static1.squarespace.com/static/5f22db0ddad7db2d2098bf70/t/624b3481b2cc8e76b88670dc/1649095821397/ActivePlus_AnnualReport_2021+%281%29.pdf.

[110] Tarik Kitson, Podcast recording with author, September 6, 2022.

[111] Tarik Kitson, Podcast recording with author, September 6, 2022.

[112] Kristy Ingram, "Why a Female Athlete Should Be Your Next Leader," EY, accessed December 8, 2022, https://www.ey.com/en_us/athlete-programs/why-female-athletes-should-be-your-next-leader.

[113] Wayne Moss, Podcast recording with author, November 2, 2021.

[114] Wayne Moss, Podcast recording with author, November 2, 2021.

[115] Ingram, "Why a Female Athlete Should Be Your Next Leader."

[116] Wayne Moss, Podcast recording with author, November 2, 2021.

[117] "State of Play 2021," Aspen Institute Project Play, accessed December 29, 2022, https://projectplay.org/state-of-play-2021/pandemic-trends.

[118] "State of Play 2022," Aspen Institute Project Play, accessed December 29, 2022, https://projectplay.org/state-of-play-2022/coaching-trends

[119] Jill Vialet, Podcast recording with author, March 22, 2022.

[120] Jill Vialet, Podcast recording with author, March 22, 2022.

[121] Jill Vialet, Podcast recording with author, March 22, 2022.

[122] Ellen Beate Hansen Sandseter and Leif Edward Ottesen Kennair, "Children's Risky Play from an Evolutionary Perspective: The Anti-Phobic Effects of Thrilling Experiences," *Evolutionary Psychology* 9, no. 2 (April 1, 2011), https://doi.org/10.1177/147470491100900212.

[123] "Playground-Related Injuries Treated in the Emergency Department," Children's Safety Network, accessed January 12, 2023, https://www.childrenssafetynetwork.org/infographics/playground-related-injuries-treated-emergency-department.

[124] Ellen Barry, "In Britain's Playgrounds, 'Bringing in Risk' to Build Resilience," *New York Times*, March 10, 2018, https://www.nytimes.com/2018/03/10/world/europe/britain-playgrounds-risk.html.

[125] Antonis Kambas et al., "Accident Prevention through Development of Coordination in Kindergarten Children," *Deutsche Zeitschrift Fur Sportmedizin* 55, no. 2 (April 18, 2004): 44–47. https://eurekamag.com/research/034/341/034341302.php.

[126] Philip Oltermann, "Learning the Ropes: Why Germany is Building Risk Into Its Playgrounds," The Guardian, October 24, 2021, https://www.theguardian.com/world/2021/oct/24/why-germany-is-building-risk-into-its-playgrounds.

[127] Let Grow Project, Implementation Guide for School Programs, 2020, https://letgrow.org/wp-content/uploads/2020/12/let-grow-project-implementation-guide-huodtr.pdf.

[128] Jill Vialet, Podcast recording with author, March 22, 2022.

[129] Diana Baumrind, "Effects of Authoritative Parental Control on Child Behavior," *Child Development* 37, no. 4 (December 1, 1966): 887–907, https://doi.org/10.1111/j.1467-8624.1966.tb05416.x.

[130] Eleanor Maccoby and John Martin, "Socialization in the Context of the Family: Parent-Child Interaction" in *Handbook of Child Psychology: Vol. 4. Socialization, Personality, and Social Development,* eds. P. H. Mussen and E. M. Hetherington (New York: Wiley, 1983) 1-101.

[131] Ian Janssen, "Hyper-Parenting Is Negatively Associated with Physical Activity among 7–12 Year Olds." *Preventive Medicine* 73 (April 1, 2015): 55–59, https://doi.org/10.1016/j.ypmed.2015.01.015.

ENDNOTES

[132] Erin Hennessy, et al., "Parent-Child Interactions and Objectively Measured Child Physical Activity: A Cross-Sectional Study," *International Journal of Behavioral Nutrition and Physical Activity* 7, no. 1 (January 1, 2010): 71, https://doi.org/10.1186/1479-5868-7-71.

[133] Ian Janssen, "Hyper-Parenting."

[134] Erin Hennessy, et al., "Parent-Child Interactions."

[135] Donglin Hu et al., "Factors That Influence Participation in Physical Activity in School-Aged Children and Adolescents: A Systematic Review from the Social Ecological Model Perspective." *International Journal of Environmental Research and Public Health* 18, no. 6 (March 18, 2021): 3147, https://doi.org/10.3390/ijerph18063147.

[136] Amanda Fitzgerald, Noelle Fitzgerald, and Cian Aherne. "Do Peers Matter? A Review of Peer and/or Friends' Influence on Physical Activity among American Adolescents," *Journal of Adolescence* 35, no. 4 (January 28, 2012): 941–58, https://doi.org/10.1016/j.adolescence.2012.01.002.

[137] Jeff Speck, Podcast recording with author, May 2, 2023.

[138] Jeff Speck, Podcast recording with author, May 2, 2023.

[139] Jeff Speck, Podcast recording with author, May 2, 2023.

[140] "Safe Routes," National Center for Safe Routes to School, accessed April 4, 2023, https://www.saferoutesinfo.org.

[141] "Communities Creating Safer Streets Starting Where Youth Walk and Bike," Vision Zero for Youth, accessed April 4, 2023, https://www.visionzeroforyouth.org.

[142] Noreen C. McDonald et al., "Impact of the Safe Routes to School Program on Walking and Bicycling." *Journal of the American Planning Association* 80, no. 2 (April 3, 2014): 153–67. https://doi.org/10.1080/01944363.2014.956654.

[143] Eleftheria Kontou et al., "U.S. Active School Travel in 2017: Prevalence and Correlates," *Preventive Medicine Reports* 17 (March 1, 2020): 101024, https://doi.org/10.1016/j.pmedr.2019.101024.

[144] U.S. Department of Health and Human Services. *Physical Activity Guidelines for Americans, 2nd edition*. Washington, DC: U.S. Department of Health and Human Services, 2018, https://health.gov/sites/default/files/2019-09/Physical_Activity_Guidelines_2nd_edition.pdf.

[145] David J. Hill et al., "Media Use in School-Aged Children and Adolescents." *Pediatrics* 138, no. 5 (October 21, 2016): e20162592, https://doi.org/10.1542/peds.2016-2592.

[146] Jackie Ostfeld, Podcast recording with author, September 7, 2020.

[147] Jackie Ostfeld, Podcast recording with author, September 7, 2020.

[148] Mike Rogerson et al.,"Regular Doses of Nature: The Efficacy of Green Exercise Interventions for Mental Wellbeing," *International Journal of Environmental Research and Public Health* 17, no. 5 (February 27, 2020): 1526, https://doi.org/10.3390/ijerph17051526.

[149] Jackie Ostfeld, Podcast recording with author, September 7, 2020.

[150] Neil E. Klepeis et al., "The National Human Activity Pattern Survey (NHAPS): A Resource for Assessing Exposure to Environmental Pollutants," *Journal of Exposure Science and Environmental Epidemiology* 11, no. 3 (July 1, 2001): 231–52, https://doi.org/10.1038/sj.jea.7500165.

[151] "National Health and Nutrition Examination Survey 2017-2018," Centers for Disease Control and Prevention, accessed January 19, 2023, https://wwwn.cdc.gov/nchs/nhanes/continuousnhanes/default.aspx?BeginYear=2017.

[152] Casey E. Gray et al., "What Is the Relationship between Outdoor Time and Physical Activity, Sedentary Behaviour, and Physical Fitness in Children? A Systematic Review." *International Journal of Environmental Research and Public Health* 12, no. 6 (June 8, 2015): 6455–74, https://doi.org/10.3390/ijerph120606455.

[153] Physical Activity Alliance, *The 2022 United States Report Card on Physical Activity for Children and Youth*, https://paamovewithus.org/wp-content/uploads/2022/10/2022-US-Report-Card-on-Physical-Activity-for-Children-and-Youth.pdf.

[154] "National Survey of Children's Health Interactive Data."

[155] "Safe Routes to Schools," Safe Routes to Schools Partnership, accessed January 19, 2023, https://www.saferoutespartnership.org/safe-routes-school.

[156] "National Health and Nutrition Examination Survey 2015-2016," Centers for Disease Control and Prevention, accessed February 2, 2022, https://wwwn.cdc.gov/nchs/nhanes/continuousnhanes/default.aspx?BeginYear=2015.

ENDNOTES

[157] Kontou et al., U.S. active school travel in 2017."

[158] "Safe Routes to Schools."

[159] Noreen C. McDonald et al., "Impact of the Safe Routes to School Program on Walking and Bicycling," *Journal of the American Planning Association* 80, no. 2 (April 3, 2014): 153–67, https://doi.org/10.1080/01944363.2014.956654.

[160] "Program Overview-Shared Streets and Spaces Grant Program," Mass.gov, accessed January 19, 2023, https://www.mass.gov/info-details/program-overview-shared-streets-and-spaces-grant-program.

[161] Teresa Earle, Podcast recording with author, July 5, 2020.

[162] Teresa Earle, Podcast recording with author, July 5, 2020.

[163] Teresa Earle, Podcast recording with author, July 5, 2020.

[164] Pat Rumbaugh, Podcast recording with author, November 23, 2021.

[165] Pat Rumbaugh, Podcast recording with author, November 23, 2021.

[166] Victoria Rideout et al., *The Common Sense Census: Media Use by Teens and Tweens 2021*, San Francisco, CA, Common Sense, 2022 https://www.commonsensemedia.org/sites/default/files/research/report/8-18-census-integrated-report-final-web_0.pdf.

[167] Jacqueline Kerr, Podcast recording with author, September 20, 2022.

[168] Jacqueline Kerr, Podcast recording with author, September 20, 2022.

[169] Jacqueline Kerr, Podcast recording with author, September 20, 2022.

[170] "Today's Parents Spend More Time with Their Kids Than Moms and Dads Did 50 Years Ago," UCI News, September 28, 2016, https://news.uci.edu/2016/09/28/todays-parents-spend-more-time-with-their-kids-than-moms-and-dads-did-50-years-ago.

[171] Minkin and Horowitz, "Parenting in America Today."

[172] Minkin and Horowitz, "Parenting in America Today."

www.ingramcontent.com/pod-product-compliance
Lightning Source LLC
LaVergne TN
LVHW021048100526
838202LV00079B/4810